Milestones in Drug Therapy
MDT

Series Editors

Prof. Dr. Michael J. Parnham
PLIVA
Research Institute
Prilaz baruna Filipovica 25
10000 Zagreb
Croatia

Prof. Dr. J. Bruinvels
INFARM
Sweelincklaan 75
NL-3723 JC Bilthoven
The Netherlands

Methotrexate

Edited by B. N. Cronstein and J. R. Bertino

Springer Basel AG

Editors

Professor Dr. Bruce N. Cronstein
Division of Rheumatology
New York University Medical Center
550 First Avenue
New York, NY 10016
USA

Professor Dr. Joseph R. Bertino
Programm in Molecular and
Pharmacologic Therapeutics
Memorial Sloan-Kettering Cancer
Center
1275 York Avenue
New York, NY 10021-6094
USA

Library of Congress Cataloging-in-Publication Data

Methotrexate / edited by B.N. Cronstein and J.R. Bertino.
   p. ; cm. – (Milestones in drug therapy)
   Includes bibliographical references and index.
   ISBN 978-3-0348-9573-6
   1. Methotrexate. I. Cronstein, Bruce N. II. Bertino, Joseph R. III. Series.
   [DNLM: 1. Methotrexate – pharmacology. 2. Methotrexate – therapeutic use. 3.
   Antimetabolites, Antineoplastic. 4. Neoplasms – drug therapy. QV 269 M5927 2000]
   RM666.M52 M48 2000
   615′.328 – dc21

Deutsche Bibliothek – CIP Einheitsaufnahme

Methotrexate / ed. by B.N. Cronstein and J.R. Bertino. –
Basel ; Boston ; Berlin : Birkhäuser, 2000
   (Milestones in drug therapy)
   ISBN 978-3-0348-9573-6   ISBN 978-3-0348-8452-5 (eBook)
   DOI 10.1007/978-3-0348-8452-5

© 2000 Springer Basel AG
Originally published by Birkhäuser Verlag, Basel in 2000

Printed on acid-free paper produced from chlorine-free pulp. TCF ∞

9 8 7 6 5 4 3 2 1

Contents

Preface

Although surprising, it seems fitting that a drug developed at the dawn of the era of rational drug design and therapeutics, methotrexate, should remain in common use for the therapy of so many different kinds of illnesses. Moreover, methotrexate has completely revolutionized the way in which medicine is practiced in a number of speciality areas. First developed to treat malignancies, methotrexate is now commonly used to treat gynecological problems, inflammatory arthritis, skin disease and probably other ailments as well. This work is designed to give a broad overview of the history of methotrexate's development, its prior use and its current therapeutic uses.

As discussed in Chapter I, aminopterin and methotrexate were designed to inhibit mammalian folate metabolism but the concept of folic acid antagonism was soon applied to the development of antibacterial and antiparasitic agents. Trimethoprim and sulfa drugs were among the first antibiotics developed and they also remain quite useful today for the treatment of a variety of infections.

Our understanding of methotrexate's mechanism of action in the therapy of malignant diseases, rheumatic diseases, skin diseases and gynecological diseases has changed over the years. The demonstration that methotrexate is a prodrug soon led to the discovery that the accumulation of other metabolites in methotrexate-treated cells and tissues might mediate the action of methotrexate. This concept is particularly relevant to the mechanism of action of methotrexate in the treatment of inflammatory diseases but may have wider application to methotrexate's mechanism of action in other areas as well.

Methotrexate was a revolutionary development, the first product of molecular medicine. The development of methotrexate ushered in the era of rational chemotherapy for malignancies. Later, methotrexate became the first systemic therapy for psoriasis and continues to be a safe and effective treatment for severe psoriasis. More recently, low dose methotrexate therapy has transformed the therapy of rheumatoid arthritis; there will never be a placebo-controlled trial of new agents for the treatment of rheumatoid arthritis as all new medications will be compared to methotrexate. More than half a century after its original synthesis methotrexate continues to surprise the medical community with new uses and novel mechanisms. It is likely that this versatile agent will continue to be with us during the coming age of genetic and molecular advancement as well.

Bruce N. Cronstein, MD

List of contributors

Graciela S. Alarcón, Division of Clinical Immunology and Rheumatology, The University of Alabama and Birmingham, MEB 615, 1813 6th Avenue So., Birmingham, AL 35294, USA; e-mail: graciela.alarcon@ccc.uab.edu

Joseph R. Bertino, Memorial Sloan-Kettering Cancer Center, 1275 York Avenue, New York, NY, USA

Edwin S. L. Chan, New York University School of Medicine, 550 First Avenue, New York, NY 10016, USA

Bruce N. Cronstein, New York University School of Medicine, 550 First Avenue, New York, NY 10016, USA

Richard I. Drachtman, Cancer Institute of New Jersey, 195 Little Albany Street, New Brunswick, NJ 80901, USA; e-mail: drachtri@umdnj.edu

Richard Gorlick, Department of Pediatrics, Memorial Sloan-Kettering Cancer Center, 1275 York Avenue, New York 10021, NY, USA; e-mail: gorlickr@mskcc.org

Barton A. Kamen, Cancer Institute of New Jersey, 195 Little Albany Street, New Brunswick, NJ 80901, USA; e-mail: kamenba@umdnj.edu

James O'Leary, Food and Drug Administration, Center for Drug Evaluation and Research, Division of Oncology Drug Products, HFD-150, 1451 Rockville Pike, Rockville, MD 20852, USA

Alexander Losev, Hem Onc Care, 2558 East 18 Street, Brooklyn, NY 11235, USA

Charles McDonald, Department of Dermatology, Rhode Island Hospital, Brown University, 593 Eddy St., Providence, RI 02903, USA

Sarah L. Morgan, Nutrition Sciences Department, The University of Alabama at Birmingham, Webb 212, Birmingham, Alabama, USA

Ana Monteagudo, Department of Obstetrics & Gynecology, New York University Medical Center, 550 First Avenue Rm 9N28, New York, NY 10023, USA; e-mail: montea01@popmail.med.nyu.edu

Franco M. Muggia, Kaplan Comprehensive Cancer Center, NYU Medical Center, 550 First Avenue, New York, NY 10016, USA; e-mail: muggif01@gcrc.med.nyu.edu

Ilan E. Timor-Tritsch, Department of Obstetrics & Gynecology, New York University Medical Center, 550 First Avenue Rm 9N28, New York, NY 10023, USA

Methotrexate
ed. by B.N. Cronstein und J.R. Bertino
© 2000 Birkhäuser Verlag Basel/Switzerland

Methotrexate: historical aspects

Joseph R. Bertino

Memorial Sloan-Kettering Cancer Center, New York, NY, USA

Introduction

In the early 1940s, folic acid was isolated and found to cure some patients with megaloblastic anemia that did not respond to vitamin B12. As acute leukemia in children had some morphological features that resembled megaloblastic anemia, patients with acute leukemia were treated with folic acid or folate conjugates (polyglutamated forms of folic acid). These proved ineffective and, in fact, were thought to accelerate the disease. The subsequent demonstration by Heinle and Welch [1] that a diet-induced deficiency of folic acid caused a decrease in the leukemia cell count, stimulated efforts, primarily by the Lederle group, to synthesize analogs of folic acid. One of these, aminopterin or 4-aminopterolylglutamic acid, proved to be a powerful antagonist that was shown by Farber et al. [2], in a landmark paper, to produce remissions in children with acute lymphocytic leukemia (ALL). With this discovery, and the demonstration by Huggins and Hodges that estrogens caused regressions in prostate cancer [3], and that nitrogen mustard caused regressions in patients with lymphoma [4], the modern era of chemotherapy was born in the 1940's.

Inhibition of folic acid metabolism

The effectiveness of aminopterin for the treatment of ALL and the demonstration of its potent antitumor effects in rodent tumors stimulated a search to pinpoint its mechanism of action. Soon after, work by Futterman indicated that this analog prevented the reduction of folic acid to active forms in chicken liver [5]. The enzyme dihydrofolate reductase (DHFR), responsible for this reduction of folic acid, was partially purified [6]. This work was followed by the seminal study of Osborne et al. [7] that showed that aminopterin was a powerful inhibitor of dihydrofolate reductase (previously also referred to as folic reductase, an enzyme that converted both folic acid as well as dihydrofolic acid to the coenzyme, tetrahydrofolic acid). This finding stimulated work on the isolation and characterization of this enzyme [9], and on the search for more selective antitumor inhibitors. Soon after, a new antagonist of parasitic growth, pyrimethamine, with minimal effects on mamalian tissue, was discovered by Russel and Hitchings [9] and was found to selectively inhibit the parasitic DHFR. Hitchings and co-workers then synthesized an antifolate that selectively inhibited the bacterial DHFR [10]. This drug, trimethoprim, in combination with a sulphonamide inhibitor of folic acid synthesis, has proven to be an effective treatment for various infections, especially those of the urinary tract. This ushered in a new concept in drug development, namely the isolation of inhibitors that exploit the differences in an enzyme obtained from different species [9–10].

In 1956, studies of L1210 leukemia-bearing mice showed that methotrexate, another folate analog, had a therapeutic index superior to that of aminopterin [11]; based on these studies, methotrexate supplanted aminopterin in the clinic. It is noteworthy that there have been no definitive trials comparing the therapeutic index of these two drugs in man. Recently, Kamen has reinitiated studies with aminopterin, based on studies that indicate it is transported and retained intracellularly to a greater degree than methotrexate [12].

Effectiveness of methotrexate in the cure of solid tumors

Eight years after the report by Farber et al., Li et al. reported that methotrexate, when given in maximally tolerated doses, produced complete responses in women with choriocarcinoma [13]. In a follow up study five years later, it became clear that many of these women had been cured [14]. These results stimulated and energized the further evaluation of methotrexate in malignant disease and a search for new drugs to treat cancer. Another human tumor found to be sensitive to single-agent treatment with either methotrexate or cyclophosphamide is Burkitt's Lymphoma [15]. Methotrexate has been widely evaluated as a single-agent and in combination to treat almost every human cancer [16]. Table 1 lists the tumors that are still treated with this drug.

Treatment of choriocarcinoma with methotrexate has provided us with proof of many concepts derived from animal tumor models, especially from the work of Skipper and colleagues [17, 18]. Some of these principles

Table 1. Malignancies in which methotrexate is used

Choriocarcinoma
Acute lymphocytic leukemia
Large cell lymphoma
High grade lymphoma
Head and neck cancer
Breast cancer
Bladder cancer
Osteogenic sarcoma

Table 2. Principles of chemotherapy: Lessons from the treatment of choriocarcinoma

1. The larger the tumor and the duration of the disease, the more difficult it is to cure.
2. Resistance occurs rapidly and is the reason for treatment failure.
3. 'Dose intensity' is important for cure.
4. A tumor cell marker (e.g. human chorionic gonadotrophin, HCG) is an important adjunct for following treatment.

are shown in Table 2. Two of these lessons are worthy of emphasis: drug resistance occurs rapidly if cure is not achieved (for most tumors within four to six months), and is the reason for treatment failure. Except for the treatment of acute leukemia, those diseases that we can cure with drugs may only require treatment for six months or less, e.g. Hodgkin's disease, diffuse large cell lymphoma, testicular cancer, small cell lung cancer, and certain childhood solid tumors. A second important point that has been learned from the experience with single-agent treatment of choriocarcinoma is that treatment with methotrexate is not associated with long term side effects, namely infertility and secondary malignancies, problems that may result from treatment with alkylating agents or radiation [19]. These side effects are of special concern when chemotherapeutic agents for cancer are used to treat non-malignant diseases.

Combination of methotrexate with other chemotherapeutic agents

Following the introduction of methotrexate into the clinic, other drugs were also found to be useful in the treatment of ALL, in particular 6-mercaptopurine (6MP), prednisone, and vincristine. A very important study by the Acute Leukemia B cooperative group showed that the combination of 6MP and methotrexate was better than either drug used alone [20]. When all four of these effective drugs were used in combination, e.g. the VAMP program, long term remissions and cures were obtained, but only in a minority of patients [21]. The next major advance that led to cures in 50% of the patients was the use of intrathecal methotrexate with adequate central nervous system (CNS) irradiation, for prophylaxis of sanctuary disease [22–23]. Further improvement in cure rates have been derived from optimal dosing and sequencing of these four drugs. In particular, methotrexate and 6MP are more effective if used in sequence: methotrexate – 6MP [24].

In 1977, the crystal structure of a bacterial DHFR was reported, the first pharmacologically important protein for which the crystal structure was available [25]. The crystal structures of avian and human DHFR proteins were subsequently solved [26], and with the advances in computer graphics have facilitated drug design and an understanding of catalysis. Mutations leading to decreased binding of methotrexate to DHFR have been found in resistant cell lines, and additional mutations have been generated by site-directed mutagenesis, facilitated by the knowledge of the structure of the protein [27]. In recent years, certain of these genes expressing mutant proteins have been used in a gene therapy strategy to confer resistance to methotrexate in hematopoietic cell precursors [28].

Resistance to methotrexate

A startling discovery was reported in 1978 by Schmike and coworkers [29]. In methotrexate resistant mouse tumor cell lines, gene amplification was shown to be responsible for the genetic mechanism resulting in the increased level of DHFR in these cells. This was an important finding, not only that, for the first time, the genetic basis for a phenotypic change was found, but also because it changed our thinking about the stability of the genome. Until then it had been assumed that the genome was stable. This discovery was preceded by the description, initially by Fisher [30], Hakala [31], Friedkin and others [32] that acquired resistance to methotrexate in tumor cells was often caused by an increase in the level of DHFR activity. Biedler and Spengler then found an abnormality in chromosomes in methotrexate-resistant cells with high levels of DHFR. They named these regions homogeneous or abnormal staining regions, because the banding pattern in these areas of the chromosome was lost [33]. Also in the early 1960s, we and others described an increase in DHFR that occurred in normal blood cells as well as in leukemia cells within a few days after treatment with methotrexate [34–36]. As most of this increased DHFR was found to be associated with bound methotrexate, and methotrexate was known to protect this enzyme from heat inactivation and proteolysis, we speculated that this increase was due to methotrexate protection of the enzyme from degradation [37]. Recent work has also raised the possibility that some or all of this 'induction' could be due to the ability of methotrexate to relieve the inhibition of DHFR translation caused by DHFR protein [38–39].

Many examples of amplification of other genes associated with resistance to other tight binding inhibitors of enzymes have followed these studies, indicating that gene amplification as a mechanism of drug resistance is not unique to methotrexate [40]. Cell lines with amplified genes and over-expression have been widely used for the study of gene regulation and for generation of large amounts of protein that may be co-amplified with methotrexate under methotrexate selection.

Two other additional discoveries have proven to be important in understanding intrinsic and acquired resistance to methotrexate: elucidation of the transport mechanism for methotrexate [41–42], and the realization that methotrexate is a prodrug, e.g. that it is converted to polyglutamate forms in cells, by a single enzyme, polyglutamate synthetase [43]. Recent studies (see chapter by Gorlick) in patients with ALL that acquire resistance to methotrexate have shown defects in leukemia cells that reduce the uptake of this drug [44]. Studies of methotrexate polyglutamate formation in leukemia cells from patients with myeloid leukemia have provided an explanation as to why these patients do not respond to methotrexate treat-ment, namely because their ability to generate methrotrexate polygluta-mates, and therefore to retain this drug, is impaired [45].

The use of methotrexate in non-neoplastic diseases

In 1951, Gubner reported that aminopterin suppressed the exudative and proliferative responses to the injection of formalin in the paws of rats [46]. Soon after, he and his colleagues published a report that showed that six of seven patients with active rheumatoid arthritis given aminopterin respond-ed rapidly with clinical improvement [47]. When the drug was stopped, relapse also occurred rapidly. The doses used were 1–2 mg/day with rest periods, that produced stomatitis, nausea, and diarrhea. Methotrexate eventually supplanted aminopterin for the treatment of this disease, and subsequent studies have shown that low, non-toxic doses of this drug are also effective in this disease.

Treatment of patients with psoriasis, initially with aminopterin, then also with low doses of methotrexate, was also found to be of benefit [47–48]; these studies were soon followed by widening indications for methotrexate. The finding that methotrexate inhibited the immune response also led to be treatment of autoimmune diseases (discussed elsewhere in this volume).

As in the case of malignant diseases, there has not been a comparative trial of aminopterin vs. methotrexate in non-malignant diseases, and it is possible that aminopterin may be more effective than methotrexate. With the development of other DHFR inhibitors as well as other antifolates that target other key folate requiring enzymes, in particular thymidylate synthase [49–50], the evaluation of these compounds for treatment of non-malignant diseases deserves consideration.

References

1 Heinle RW, Welch AD (1948) Experiments with pteroylglutamic acid and pteroylglutamic acid deficiency in human leukemia. *J Clin Invest* 27: 539 (Abstr)
2 Farber S, Diamond LK, Mercer RD, Sylvester RF Jr, Wolf JA (1948) Temporary remissions in acute leukemia in children produced by folic acid antagonist, 4-aminopteroyl-glutamic acid (aminopterin). *N Engl J Med* 238: 787–793
3 Huggins C, Hodges CV (1941) Studies on prostate cancer: Effects of castration on advanced carcinoma of the prostate gland. *Arch Surg* 43: 209–223
4 Gilman A (1963) The initial clinical trial of nitrogen mustard. *Am J Surg* 105: 574–578
5 Futterman S (1957) Enzymatic Reduction of folic acid and dihydrofolic acid to tetrahydro-folic acid. *J Biol Chem* 228: 1031–1038

6 Perkins JP, Hillcoat BL, Bertino JR (1967) Dihydrofolate reductase from a resistant subline of the L1210 lymphoma. Purification and properties. *J Biol Chem* 242: 4771–4776

7 Osborne MJ, Freeman M, Huennekens FM (1958) Inhibition of dihydrofolic reductase by aminopterin and amethopterin. *Proc Soc Exp Biol Med* 97: 429–431

8 Huennekens FM (1996) In search of dihydrofolate reductase. *Protein Science* 5: 1201–1208

9 Hitchings GH (1989) Selective inhibitors of dihydrofolate reductase. (Nobel Lecture in physiology or medicine, 1988) *In Vitro Cell Dev Biol* 25: 303–310

10 Hitchings GH, Burchall JJ, Ferone R (1966) The comparative enzymology of dihydrofolate reductase and the design of chemotherapeutic agents. *Symp Soc Gen Microbiol* 16: 294–301

11 Goldin A (1968) Preclinical methodology for the selection of anticancer agents. In: H Busch (ed): *Methods in Cancer Research*, vol IV., Academic Press, New York, NY, 193–254

12 Smith A, Hum M, Winick NJ, Kamen BA (1996) A case for the use of aminopterin in treatment of patients with leukemia based on metabolic studies of blasts *in vitro*. *Clin Cancer Res* 2: 69–73

13 Li MC, Hertz R, Spencer DB (1956) Effect of methotrexate therapy upon choriocarcinoma and chorioadenoma. *Proc Soc Exp Biol Med* 93: 361–366

14 Hertz R, Lewis J Jr, Lipsett MB (1961) Five years experience with the chemotherapy of metastatic choriocarcinoma and related trophoblastic tumors in women. *Am J Obstet Gynecol* 82: 631–637

15 Oettgen HF, Burkitt D, Burchenal JH (1963) Malignant lymphoma involving the jaw in African children. Treatment with methotrexate. *Cancer* 16: 616–621

16 Bertino JR (1993) Karnofsky Memorial Lecture. Ode tomethotrexate. *J Clin Oncol* 11: 5–14

17 Skipper HE, Schabel FM Jr, Wilcox WAS (1964) Experimental evaluation of potential anti-cancer agents. XIII. On the criteria and kinetics associated with curability of experimental leukemia. *Cancer Chemother Rep* 35: 1–15

18 Skipper HE, Schabel FM Jr (1982) Quantitative and cytokinetic studies in experimental tumor systems. In: Holland JF, Frei E III (eds): *Cancer Medicine*. Lea & Febiger, Philadelphia, PA, 663–672

19 Rustin GJS, Rustin F, Dent J, Booth H, Sah S, Bagshaw KU (1983) No increase in second tumors after cytotoxic chemotherapy for gestational neoplasms. *N Engl J Med* 308: 1–5

20 Acute Leukemia Group B (1961) Studies of sequential and combination antimetabolite therapy in acute leukemia: 6-Mercaptopurine and methotrxate. *Blood* 18: 431–441

21 Freireich EJ, Karon M, Frei E III (1964) Quadruple combination therapy (VAMP) for acute lymphocytic leukemia. *Proc Am Assoc Cancer Res* 5: 20 (Abstr)

22 Aur RJA, Simone J, Husta HO, Verzosa MS (1971) Central nervous system therapy and combination chemotherapy in childhood lymphocytic leukemia. *Blood* 37: 272–275

23 Simone JV, Aur RJA, Husta HD, Verzosa MS (1978) Three to ten years after cessation of therapy in children with leukemia. *Cancer* 42: 839–844

24 Camitta B, Levanthal B, Lauer S, Shuster JJ, Adair S, Casper J, Civin C, Graham M, Mahoney D, Munoz L, Kamen B, Manoza H, Keiser G, Kam G (1989) Intermediate-dose intravenous methotrexate and mercaptopurine therapy for non-T non-B acute lymphocytic leukemia of childhood: A Pediatric Oncology Group Study. *J Clin Oncol* 7: 1539–1544

25 Matthews DP, Alden RA, Bolin JT, Freer ST, Hemlin R, Xyong N, Kraut S, Poe M, Williams M, Hoogsteen K (1977) Dihydrofolate reductase: X-ray structure of the binary complex with methotrexate. Science 197: 452–455

26 Oefner C, D'Arcy A, Winkler FK (1988) Crystal structure of human dihydrofolate reductase complexed with folate. *Eur J Biochem* 174: 377–385

27 Schweitzer BI, Dicker AP, Bertino JR (1990) Dihydrofolate reductase as a therapeutic target. FASEB J 4: 2441–2452

28 Banerjee D, Zhao SC, Li MX, Schweitzer BI, Mineishi S, Bertino JR (1994) Gene Therapy utilizing drug resistance genes: a review. *Stem Cells* 12: 378–385

29 Alt FW, Kellems RE, Bertino JR, Schimke RT (1978) Selective multiplication of dihydro-folate reductase genes in methotrexate resistant variants of cultured murine cells. *J Biol Chem* 253: 1357–1370

30 Fisher GA (1961) Increased levels of folic acid reductase as a mechanism of resistance to methopterin in leukemic cells. *Biochem Pharmacol* 7: 75–77

31 Hakala MT, Zakrewski SF, Nichol CA (1961) Relation of folic acid reductase to ame-thopterin resistance in cultured mammalian cells. *J Biol Chem* 236: 952–958

32 Friedkin M, Crawford E, Humphreys SR, Goldin A (1962) The association of increased dihydrofolate reductase with amethopterin resistance in mouse leukemia. *Cancer Res* 22: 600–606

33 Biedler JL, Spengler B (1976) Metaphase chromosome anomaly: Association with drug resistance and cell specific products. *Science* 191: 185–187

34 Bertino JR (1963) The mechanism of action of the folate antagonists in man. *Cancer Res* 23: 1286–1306

35 Bertino JR, Cashmore A, Fink M, Calabresi P, Lefkowitz E (1965) The induction of leukocyte and erythrocyte dihydrofolate reductase by methotrexate. II. Clinical and pharmacologic studies. *Clin Pharmacol Ther* 6: 763–770

36 Bertino JR, Donohue DR, Simmons B (1963) Induction of dihydrofolate reductase activity in leukocytes and erythrocytes of patients treated with amethopterin. *J Clin Invest* 42: 466–475

37 Hillcoat BL, Sweet V, Bertino JR (1967) Increase of dihydrofolate reductase activity in cultured mammalian cells after exposure to methotrexate. *Proc Natl Acad Sci USA* 58: 1632–1637

38 Chu E, Koeller DM, Casey JL, Drake JC, Chabner BA, Elwood PC, Zinn S, Allegra G (1991) Autoregulation of human thymidylate messenger RNA translation by thymidylate synthase. *Proc Natl Acad Sci USA* 88: 8977–8981

39 Abali-Ercikan EA, Banerjee D, Waltham MC, Skacel N, Scotto KW, Bertino JR (1997) Dihydrofolate reductase protein inhibits its own translation by binding to dihydrofolate reductase mRNA sequences within the coding region. *Biochemistry* 36: 12317–12322

40 Dube S, Bertino JR (1991) Gene amplification. In: R Dulbecco (ed): *Encyclopedia of Human Biology.* Academic Press, San Diego, CA, 785–789

41 Sirotnak FM (1980) Correlates of folate analog transport, pharmacokinetics and selective antitumor action. *Pharmacol Ther* 8: 71–104

42 Jansen G (1998) Receptor and carrier-mediated transport systems for folates and antifolates. In: A Jackman (ed): *Anticancer Drug Development Guide: Antifolate Drugs in Cancer Therapy.* Hulmana Press Inc., Totana, NJ 293–321

43 Chabner BA, Allegra CA, Curt GA, Cleudeniun NJ, Baram J, Koizumi S, Drake K, Jolivet J (1985) Polyglutamylation of methotrexate: Is methotrexate a prodrug? *J Clin Invest* 76: 907–912

44 Gorlick R, Goker E, Trippett T, Waltham M, Banerjee D, Bertino JR (1996) Drug Therapy: Intrinsic and acquired resistance to methotrexate in acute leukemia. *NEJM* 335: 1041–1048

45 Lin JT, Tong WP, Trippett TM, Niedznieki D, Tao T, Tan C, Steinherz P, Schweitzer BI, Bertino JR (1991) Basis for natural resistance to methotrexate in human acute nonlymphocytic leukemia. *Leukemia Res* 15: 1191–1196

46 Gubner R (1951) Therapeutic suppression of tissue reactivity. I. Comparison of the effects of cortisone and aminopterin. *Amer J Med Sc* 221: 169–175

47 Gubner R (1951) Therapeutic suppression of tissue reactivity. II. Effect of aminopterin in rheumatoid arthritis and psoriasis. *Amer J Med Sc* 221: 176–182

48 McDonald CJ (1997) Hyperproliferative skin diseases. In: CJ McDonald (ed): *Immunomodulartory and Cytotoxic Agents in Dermatology.* Marcel Dekker, Inc., NY, 267–282

49 Jackman AL, Calvert AH (1995) Folate-based thymdylate synthase inhibitor as anticancer drugs. *Ann Oncol* 6: 871–881

50 Rutin Y, Haistick A CAOS, Vanhoefer U, Yin MB, Wilke H, Seeber S (1991) Thymdylate synthase inhibitors in cancer therapy: direct and indirect inhibitors. *J Clin Oncol* 15: 389–400

Methotrexate
ed. by B. N. Cronstein und J. R. Bertino
© 2000 Birkhäuser Verlag Basel/Switzerland

Methotrexate, its mechanism of action in malignant disease and mechanisms of resistance by malignant cells

Richard Gorlick

*Department of Pediatrics, Memorial Sloan-Kettering Cancer Center, 1275 York Avenue,
New York, USA*

Introduction

Methotrexate (MTX), an antifolate inhibitor of dihydrofolate reductase (DHFR), is used widely, as described in Chapters IV and V, for the treatment of various forms of cancer, such as lymphoma, acute lymphocytic leukemia (ALL), germ cell tumors, breast cancer, gastric cancer, bladder cancer, osteogenic sarcoma (OS), and head and neck cancer [1], Aminopterin, an antifolate now supplanted by MTX, was the first drug capable of inducing complete remissions in children with ALL [2]. MTX administered as a single agent at maximally tolerated doses was one of the first agents shown to be capable of curing a human malignancy (choriocarcinoma) [3]. Although dramatic responses and even cure are observed in some of these malignancies with MTX treatment alone or in combination, in the majority of tumors such as acute myelocytic leukemia (AML), intrinsic resistance effectively prevents the use of this agent. In malignancies which are initially sensitive to therapy, e.g. ALL, acquired resistance may develop contributing to treatment failure and relapse [4].

MTX is an ideal drug for studying mechanisms of action and resistance as its intracellular metabolism and targets, in tumors, have been well characterized. Over the past decade many of the genes involved in folate metabolism have been cloned. This information coupled with the development of new sensitive molecular biology techniques, has made it possible to identify and study the changes associated with intrinsic and acquired resistance to MTX in tumors from patients. In addition, this information has facilitated more in depth studies of folate and antifolate metabolism. In this chapter the mechanism of action of the antifolates, focusing on newer insights into its metabolism, will be reviewed. Studies of the mechanisms of intrinsic and acquired resistance to MTX observed in tumor samples obtained from patients will also be described.

Mechanism of methotrexate action

MTX is cytotoxic to tumor cells through inhibiting enzymes needed to produce essential cofactors for nucleotide biosynthesis, particularly thymidine. Rapidly dividing tumor cells, when depleted of these nucleotides, essential for DNA synthesis and cell division, are killed presumably through apoptotic pathways [5, 6]. The metabolism of MTX intracellularly is an important determinant of its cytotoxicity.

Although MTX action is understood in considerable detail, we continue to learn more about this drug in relation to folate metabolism. MTX, being a structural analogue of folic acid, is metabolized intracellularly in a similar manner to the normal folate substrates (Fig. 1) [1, 6]. MTX enters cells through a carrier transport mechanism used by reduced folates, by binding to folate receptors (FR) and entering through an endocytic pathway, or potentially through other transporters with different physiological properties [7–11]. Once inside the cell, MTX is polyglutamylated,

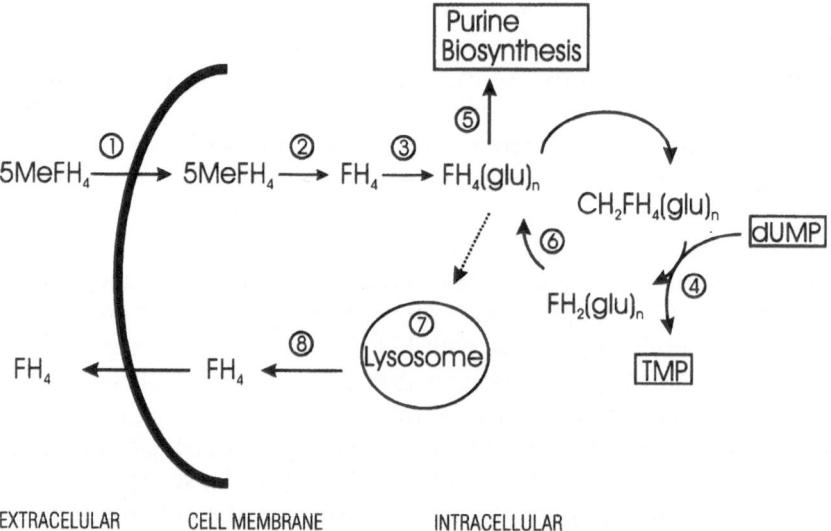

EXTRACELULAR   CELL MEMBRANE   INTRACELLULAR

Figure 1. Normal folate metabolism. 5-methyltetrahydrofolate ($5MeFH_4$) is the major physiological serum folate in humans. It is transported into mammalian cells by the reduced folate carrier, an endocytic pathway activated by a folate receptor or potentially through a folate transporter (1). Once inside the cell $5MeFH_4$ is converted to tetrahydrofolate (FH_4) by the enzyme methionine synthase which also generates methionine from homocysteine (2). FH_4 is polyglutamylated by the enzyme folylpolyglutamate synthetase (3). FH_4 is converted to 5,10-methylenetetrahydrofolate (CH_2FH_4) which is an essential cofactor for thymidylate synthase (4). Thymidylate synthase produces thymidine monophosphate (TMP) from deoxyuridine monophosphate (dUMP). Both FH_4 and CH_2FH_4 can be converted to 10-formyl tetrahydrofolate which is an essential cofactor for two enzymes involved in purine biosynthesis (5). Dihydrofolate reductase is the only enzyme capable of regenerating FH_4 from dihydrofolate (FH_2) (6). FH_4 polyglutamates are transported into and hydrolyzed in the lysosome to monoglutamate forms by the enzyme gamma glutamyl hydrolase (7). Free FH_4 is rapidly effluxed through an energy dependent transporter (8).

i.e. additional glutamates (up to five) are added via linkage to the γ-carboxyl of glutamate. MTX polyglutamates are retained for longer periods in cells compared to MTX, as free MTX is actively effluxed. MTX and MTX polyglutamates bind tightly but reversibly to the enzyme DHFR, thus inhibiting tetrahydrofolate formation, required for thymidylate bio-synthesis [4]. In addition, MTX polyglutamates as well as dihydrofolate polyglutamates (the latter accumulated due to DHFR inhibition) inhibit the enzymes of purine synthesis, including 5′-phosphoribosylglycinamide (GAR) and aminoimidazole carboxamide ribonucleotide (AICAR) trans-formylases [12, 13]. MTX is cytotoxic to tumors during the S phase of the cell cycle when purines and pyrimidines are required for DNA synthesis.

Methotrexate Transport

Folates, in their monoglutamate forms, can be transported into cells via multiple pathways. These include the reduced folate carrier (RFC), an endocytic mechanism termed 'potocytosis' which requires binding to a glycosylphosphatidylinositol anchored FR in cell membranes, or through a more recently identified low pH folate transporter [10, 11, 14, 15]. The FR and RFC are expressed at different levels in different tissues with some cells, such as leukemic blasts, expressing both proteins. The RFC has the properties of a bidirectional anion exchanger and does not hydrolyze ATP as part of its function. It has a high turnover number and a higher affinity for MTX and reduced folates (1–5 μM) than for folic acid (100–200 μM) [16]. The cDNA for the RFC has recently been identified in hamster, mouse, and human cells [17–22]. In contrast to the RFC, the FR are low capacity transporters with a high affinity for folic acid (1 nM) and the reduced folates 5-formyl and 5-methyltetrahydrofolate (10–40 nM) and a lower affinity for MTX and other 4-amino-antifolates (0.15–1.7 μM) [16]. Three folate receptor genes have been cloned to date (α, β, and γ). The distribution of this protein(s), as studied by immunohistochemistry, is limited to a few normal tissues that include the kidney tubules and the choroid plexus [23]. Its function may be to conserve or partition folates in specific tissues. Certain tumors, especially ovarian cancer, have high levels of this protein [24]. In cell lines expressing both the FR and the RFC, over-all drug sensitivity to MTX and certain other folate antagonists appeared to correlate with differential efficacy of drug transport via the RFC rather than by the FR [16, 25]. Recently, Goldman et al. have reported the presence of a third transport route which has its maximal activity at a low pH [10, 11]. This may be of importance in the transport of folates across the epithelia of the small intestine. At present, transport of folates through this route has only been demonstrated in a murine leukemia cell line with abnormal RFC function and Chinese hamster ovary cells selected for resistance with a lipophilic antifolate (pyrimethamine) [10, 11, 26]. The physiological role and genetic origin of this transporter remain unclear. Work by Goldman et al. has demonstrated that the MTX efflux pathway may also be an important determinant of the intracellular levels of free monoglutamyl folates within the cell [27, 28]. The Chinese hamster ovary cell line selected using pyrimethamine was also resistant to other lipophilic antifolates based on a loss of folate export function. Loss of the folate exporter led to resistance through an expansion of the folate pool size [11]. The efflux pathway may be particularly important in determining equilibrium folate levels as the efflux pathway is energy dependent, in contrast to the predominant influx pathway [27, 28]. The genetic identity of the folate exporter is unknown but it is postulated to be a member of the multispecific organic-anion transporter (MOAT) or multi-drug resistance associated protein (MRP) family [29].

Methotrexate polyglutamylation

Intracellular MTX polyglutamates are generated by the enzyme folylpolyglutamate synthetase (FPGS) whereas catabolism of MTX polyglutamates is dependent on the rates of entry of polyglutamates into lysosomes and hydrolysis by the lysosomal enzyme gamma-glutamyl hydrolase (GGH) [30]. Mammalian FPGS is a well characterized mitochondrial and cytoplasmic enzyme that catalyzes the sequential ATP-dependent addition of glutamates to all naturally occurring folates as well as many folate analogs including MTX [31]. FPGS has a higher affinity for naturally occurring folates as compared to MTX, therefore changes in FPGS activity have a more profound affect on MTX polyglutamylation and its cytotoxicity than on folate pool size [6]. The cDNA encoding this gene has been identified [32]. Studies have further elucidated the genomic organization of the gene encoding this enzyme and have identified numerous splice variants in the mouse and human FPGS gene [33–35]. Recent studies have characterized the promoter region and the transcriptional regulation of this gene [36] and these suggest that there may be differences in the kinetic properties of FPGS in different cell types [37].

Compared to FPGS, less is known about GGH. While it is generally accepted that the predominant lysosomal enzyme form is the most important in regulation of folate and antifolate polyglutamate chain length, the content and specificity of the enzyme varies markedly across cell types, tissues, and different species [38]. For example, GGH from rodent cultured cells is primarily an endopeptidase (cleaving the innermost γ-linkage) [39, 40], while the enzyme from human sarcoma cells (HT-1080) displays almost exclusive exopeptidase (cleaving the last or penultimate γ-linkage) activity under identical conditions [41]. It is not clearly understood but the majority of GGH in cell lines is constitutively secreted. The recent identification of the cDNA for rat and human GGH may allow a determination of the role of GGH [42, 43]. Glutamine antagonists which are inhibitors of human GGH, such as 6-diazo-5-oxo-L-norleucine (DON) have been identified and may aid in elucidating the role of GGH in MTX metabolism [41].

Translational autoregulation

Administration of MTX to patients leads to an increase in the level of DHFR protein (mostly bound to MTX) in both normal and leukemic leukocytes as well as in erythrocytes within hours to days [44]. *In vitro* studies using an ALL cell line showed that the increase in DHFR protein was not inhibited by actinomycin D, but was abrogated by cycloheximide treatment, suggesting that the increase was not due to increased transcription. The rapid increase in DHFR observed after MTX treatment could not be explained either by protection of DHFR from degradation by bound MTX and/or dihydrofolate or by new protein synthesis [44]. An analogous increase in thymidylate synthase (TS) activity has been reported to occur in tumor cells after 5-fluorouracil treatment, and it has been suggested that this increase may be due to regulation at the translational level [45]. Studies *in vitro* using a rabbit reticulocyte translation system have shown that DHFR protein inhibits its own synthesis [46]. The reversal of this inhibition by MTX or dihydrofolate may in part explain the observed increase in DHFR activity in normal and leukemic cells after MTX treatment [46]. Recent studies have revealed that a small region towards the 3' end of its coding region may be involved in the binding [47]. The relationship between this increase in DHFR protein after MTX administration and resistance to MTX is not clear.

Resistance mechanisms to methotrexate in experimental tumors

Knowledge of the mechanisms of MTX action and its metabolism has allowed the elucidation of various mechanisms by which cells acquire resistance to MTX (Tab. 1) [1]. Two common mechanisms of MTX resistance found in experimental tumors are an increase in DHFR enzyme activity due to gene amplification and a decrease in drug transport [1, 4]. When DHFR gene amplification occurs as a result of stepwise MTX selection the genetic reduplication can take the form of a homogeneously staining region or occur on non integrated pieces of DNA, referred to as double-minute chromosomes, or on submicroscopic elements referred to as amplisomes [6]. Heterogeneous staining regions appear to confer stable drug resistance whereas double-minute chromosomes and amplisomes revert to the wild type phenotype when the selective pressure is removed [6]. Decreased MTX transport in the majority of cell lines is associated

Table 1. Mechanisms of resistance to methotrexate in experimental systems

Mechanism of resistance	Cellular alteration resulting in resistance
Decreased drug influx	Decreased RFC expression Mutations in RFC which change function
Increased folate pools	Mutations in RFC which change affinity Decrease in folate efflux
Decreased polyglutamylation	Decreased FPGS expression Decreased FPGS affinity for binding substrates Increased GGH expression
Increased DHFR activity	DHFR gene amplification Increased DHFR transcription (cell cycle related genes) Increased DHFR translation (translational autoregulation)
Decreased DHFR affinity	Mutations in DHFR
Increased use of nucleotide salvage pathways	Unknown

Abbreviations used: RFC, reduced folate carrier; FPGS, folylpolyglutamate synthetase; GGH, gamma-glutamyl hydrolase; DHFR, dihydrofolate reductase.

with decreased RFC expression [48]. Cell lines with mutations in the RFC that are associated with decreased MTX transport have been reported [49, 50].

Less commonly, a decrease in retention of MTX due to defective polyglutamylation, a decrease in binding of MTX to DHFR, changes in folate pool size, or increased use of salvage pathways have been associated with MTX resistance in cell lines [51–56]. In addition, model systems have shown that translational autoregulation and alterations in genes associated with cell cycle regulation, by influencing DHFR transcription, may result in MTX resistance [1, 47]. Defective polyglutamylation resulting in MTX resistance has been associated with both decreases in FPGS activity as well as increases in GGH activity [51, 57]. Resistance to MTX based on defective polyglutamylation is schedule dependent, in contrast, to changes in transport or DHFR which are more dose dependent [1, 4]. Changes in the binding affinity of DHFR for MTX as a substrate are the result of mutations in the DHFR gene [56]. A number of these mutations have been described and well characterized. These mutations frequently are selective and have minimal effects on the binding of dihydrofolate to DHFR [56]. Increases in folate pool sizes have also been shown to be associated with MTX resistance in cell lines. Increased folate pools compete with MTX more effectively for the enzymes involved in folate metabolism including FPGS and DHFR. An L1210 murine leukemia cell line selected for resistance to lometrexol (DDATHF) became cross-resistant to many antifolates because of an expanded folate pool [52]. The expanded folate pool in this cell line was the result of two mutations in the RFC, which preserved its function while making folic acid the preferred substrate [52]. An expanded folate pool was also the mechanism of resistance in the cell line described previously with decreased folate efflux [11]. Finally, because antifolates are cytotoxic to cells through depletion of intracellular nucleotides, utilization of an alternative pathway for their synthesis can lead to resistance. Inhibition of the *de novo* synthesis pathways by antifolates can at least partly be compensated for through utilization of the salvage pathway [53–55]. In fibroblast and human hematologic cell lines it has been shown that the addition of a nucleoside transport inhibitor which blocks the salvage pathway, such as dipyridamole, enhances the cytotoxicity of MTX [53, 54]. This finding suggests that the salvage pathway may play a role in MTX resistance.

With an understanding of the mechanism of action of MTX and resistance mechanisms in experimental systems, as well as sensitive techniques to measure these events, attention has now focused on tumor samples from patients to determine the mechanisms of acquired and intrinsic resistance to MTX. The acute leukemias have been the initial focus of research because relatively pure populations of tumor cells can easily be obtained. Leukemic blasts obtained from patients with AML at diagnosis can be considered intrinsically resistant, as the single-agent response rate to MTX in this disease is approximately 15%, and MTX is not a routine component of therapy [1]. In contrast, ALL is sensitive to antifolates with MTX remaining a major component of therapy particularly during the maintenance phase of treatment. When patients with ALL relapse after having received MTX treatment their blasts can be studied for mechanisms of acquired MTX resistance [1]. In the following sections the mechanisms of MTX resistance in leukemia samples and solid tumors will be reviewed.

Intrinsic resistance to methotrexate

Leukemic blast cells obtained from patients with untreated AML and its subtypes provide an opportunity to investigate mechanisms of intrinsic MTX resistance. After an *in vitro* 24 hour incubation with [³H]-MTX, MTX polyglutamates were separated by high pressure liquid chromatography (HPLC) and the radioactivity was quantitated with a scintillation counter in blasts from 43 patients with AML and the results compared to blasts from 34 patients with pediatric pre B ALL. The AML blasts, as compared to the ALL blasts, were less able to form long chain polyglutamates (Fig. 2) [58–60]. Studies were also performed with these blast cells to detect other possible mechanisms of MTX resistance. Transport resistance was relatively uncommon in AML and no evidence for either increases in DHFR activity or alterations in DHFR were found. The basis for the intrinsic resistance of AML to MTX therefore appears to be predominantly due to impaired polyglutamylation. This conclusion supports a previous study that showed that there was no difference in inhibition of DNA bio-

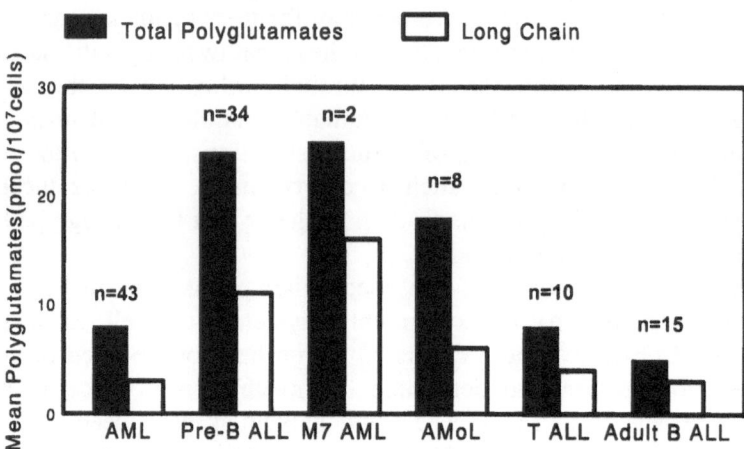

Figure 2. Total MTX polyglutamates and long chain MTX polyglutamates (glu$_{3-6}$) in leukemic blasts obtained from untreated patients with acute myelocytic leukemia (AML), pediatric pre-B acute lymphocytic leukemia (ALL), AML (M7 subtype), acute monocytic leukemia (AMoL, M5 subtype), T cell ALL, and adult B cell ALL.

synthesis in AML vs. ALL cells by MTX after short term incubations with this drug [61]. However, polyglutamylation defects are noted if the cells are then washed free of extracellular MTX and inhibition of thymidylate or DNA synthesis is measured several hours later [62].

Intrinsic MTX resistance was studied in soft tissue sarcoma and epidermoid carcinoma and, in most samples, may result from impaired polyglutamylation. In a study of fifteen soft tissue sarcoma samples, ten of the twelve which were resistant to MTX had markedly decreased long chain polyglutamate formation. Intrinsic defects in MTX transport were not observed but, in contrast to AML, DHFR amplification was observed in four of the eight samples tested [63]. In a study of cervical and head and neck squamous cell carcinoma cell lines, intrinsic resistance to MTX was found to be secondary to impaired polyglutamylation. No alterations in MTX transport or DHFR levels were observed [64, 65].

The ability of blasts to form significant amounts of long chain MTX polyglutamates has been identified as an important determinant of the outcome of ALL treatment. Adult T lineage as well as adult B lineage ALL were compared to pediatric B lineage ALL and both adult groups were found to accumulate lower amounts of long chain polyglutamates, correlating with prognosis (Fig. 2) [59]. Pediatric T lineage ALL blasts compared to B lineage ALL blasts were also found to accumulate significantly less long chain polyglutamates [59, 66]. Hyperdiploid B lineage blasts were found to accumulate significantly more long chain polyglutamates, once again correlating with a favorable outcome [67]. The ability of leukemia blasts to accumulate MTX and MTX polyglutamates was tested as a prognostic factor at diagnosis in childhood ALL. Children whose lymphoblasts simultaneously accumulated both high MTX and high MTX polyglutamate levels had a significantly better event-free survival than those who accumulated either low MTX or low MTX polyglutamates or both (65% ± 15% vs. 22% ± 9%, p = 0.01). These correlations were observed only in "good" but not "poor risk" subgroups [68]. This study demonstrated that even in "good risk" ALL patients, there may be some whose blasts form low levels of MTX polyglutamates, and may have a poor prognosis. However, to date, polyglutamylation of MTX as an independent variable has not been evaluated.

Of interest is that two subsets of AML (FAB classifications – M5 and M7 subtypes) have been found to accumulate MTX polyglutamates, following *in vitro* exposure to [^{3}H]-MTX, to almost the same levels as childhood ALL blasts [60, 69]. It may be worthwhile testing MTX for efficacy in these AML subtypes as the value of this drug in treating these AML subsets may have been overlooked because of the relative rarity of these diseases.

Studies are beginning to clarify the relative contributions that alterations of FPGS and GGH activities and transport of MTX polyglutamates into lysosomes provide to MTX resistance due to decreased polyglutamate accumulation. Studies have shown higher FPGS activities in B lineage ALL as compared to T lineage ALL blasts, consistent with the differences observed in intracellular levels of MTX polyglutamates measured after incubation with tritiated MTX [66, 70]. These studies failed to show a direct correlation between FPGS activity and MTX polyglutamylation. Recent studies have shown that the ratio of FPGS/GGH enzyme activity correlates with MTX polyglutamylation [30, 71]. It is therefore a combination of both activities which likely determines the level of MTX polyglutamylation in a cell. The recent cloning of the cDNA's encoding GGH and FPGS will allow quantitation of the expression of these genes; a quantitative reverse transcription PCR methodology for measuring FPGS and GGH mRNA expression in leukemic blasts has recently been developed [32, 43, 72].

Another potential basis for the differences in polyglutamylation between intrinsically MTX sensitive and resistant tumors, which requires further study, is the possibility that different isoforms of FPGS are expressed in different tissues. A recent study has shown a two-fold difference in the affinity (K_m) for MTX between AML and ALL cell lines and blast samples [37]. A previous study of soft tissue sarcoma cell lines had also shown a difference in the K_m of FPGS for MTX in resistant as compared to MTX sensitive cell lines [63]. Selective expression of different splice variants in different tissues may explain this observation, but further studies will be necessary to determine if different isoforms of FPGS are expressed in different cell types.

Acquired resistance to methotrexate

Transport defects

Standard radiolabeled transport assays have played a limited role in the assessment of transport defects in the clinical setting due to the inability to obtain an adequate sample size and the difficulty interpreting data accurately due to heterogeneity within the sample. In an effort to overcome these limitations, a competitive displacement flow cytometric assay utilizing the fluorescent lysine analog of MTX, N^{α}-(4-amino-4-deoxy-N^{10}-methylpteroyl)-N^{ϵ}-(4'-fluoresceinthiocarbamyl)-L-lysine or PT-430, was developed as a sensitive method for the detection of transport resistance to MTX in blast cells obtained from leukemia patients [73]. The essential component of the assay, PT-430, is rapidly taken up into blasts utilizing a different transport mechanism to that of MTX and binds directly to DHFR; thus making it an effective intracellular marker. After achievement of steady-state levels of intracellular PT-430, subsequent incubation with the competitors, MTX and trimetrexate (TMTX) which differ in the mode of carrier transport, produces characteristic displacement patterns of PT-430 distinguishing MTX transport defective blasts from those with normal transport [73]. MTX transport was examined in 27 patients with untreated ALL and 31 patients with relapsed ALL using this assay. Only 13% of untreated patients were considered to have impaired MTX transport whereas more than 70% of relapsed patients had evidence of impaired MTX transport, indicating that decreased transport is a common acquired resistance mechanism to MTX in relapsed ALL [73, 74]. Of interest, in newly diagnosed AML patients analyzed by this assay a heterogeneous pattern was observed with variable displacement seen with MTX as well as TMTX. A subset of patients were found to have minimal uptake of TMTX suggesting resistance to this agent. A possible explanation for this observation is the expression of p-glycoprotein, the product of the multi-drug resistance (MDR) gene in these cells, which has been described in newly diagnosed patients with AML and can result in the efflux of trimetrexate [74].

The availability of cDNA clones encoding the human RFC has allowed studies of the molecular basis of impaired MTX transport. A quantitative RT-PCR methodology was developed to measure RFC mRNA expression. Of nine transport-defective ALL samples, five had decreased and one had no detectable RFC expression. In the remaining three samples the basis of the impaired transport was unclear, and may be due to mutations in the RFC gene [74]. Mutations in the RFC gene resulting in decreased MTX transport have been described in mouse and human leukemia cell lines [49, 50]. In another study RFC mRNA expression as measured by RT-PCR was related to [^{3}H]-MTX uptake in pediatric ALL. The RFC expression was much more predictive of MTX transport in B-precursor as compared to

T-precursor ALL. Hyperdiploidy in B-precursor ALL, with increased copies of chromosome 21 (the chromosomal location of the RFC gene), was associated with increased RFC transcripts [75]. It was postulated that the good prognosis of children with hyperdiploid B-precursor ALL treated with antimetabolites may reflect increased RFC expression and capacities for MTX transport [75].

DHFR gene amplification

A common mechanism of resistance to MTX in many experimental tumors is an increase in DHFR activity due to gene amplification [76]. Resistance to MTX in mouse, hamster, and human cell lines grown in sequentially increased MTX concentrations has been shown in most cases to be due to increased DHFR synthesis and a proportional increase in DHFR gene copy number [77, 78]. Four case reports appeared subsequently in the literature, indicating that low level gene amplification occurs in tumor cells from patients treated with MTX, consistent with the expectation that a low level amplification would be sufficient to cause clinical resistance to this drug [56]. Based on these findings, leukemic blasts from 29 patients with relapsed ALL who had been treated with MTX were analyzed using a sensitive dot blot assay; low level (2–4 copy number) DHFR gene amplification was detected in approximately 30% of samples (9 out of 29 samples). In contrast gene amplification was present in only four of the 38 samples of leukemic blasts obtained from patients with newly diagnosed ALL and in one of the 53 samples of leukemic blasts obtained from patients with newly diagnosed AML. The results of the dot blot assays were confirmed by Southern and Northern analysis, as well as DHFR enzyme activity in several cases [79]. DHFR gene amplification is a frequent mechanism of acquired resistance to MTX, occurring in approximately 20–30% of relapsed ALL patients. In some patient samples, as has been observed in experimental tumors made resistant to MTX, both impaired transport and increased DHFR activity were observed.

The amount and heterogeneity of expression of DHFR in ALL blast cells has also been analyzed at diagnosis and relapse in ALL samples, utilizing a PT-430 assay [80]. At initial diagnosis 30 of the 45 T-cell ALL samples (78%) exhibited dual blast populations with one population 'exhibiting' higher levels of DHFR as measured by higher levels of PT 430 fluorescence. In B-cell ALL specimens 17 of the 36 samples (47%) exhibited dual populations [80]. Heterogeneous DHFR expression therefore correlated more closely with a T cell ALL phenotype which has been associated with a worse prognosis. For patients with low white blood cell (WBC) counts (< 50,000) at presentation with ALL the presence of DHFR overexpression was associated with a decreased event-free survival ($p < 0.016$), a relationship not observed in patients with high WBC counts at presentation.

At relapse, 11 of 14 samples exhibited dual blast populations [80]. This study suggests that marked heterogeneity exists in leukemic blasts for DHFR levels, and high levels of DHFR at diagnosis and relapse may be an important and clinically relevant mechanism of intrinsic and acquired resistance to MTX in ALL [80].

DHFR mutations

Mutations in the DHFR gene, resulting in an altered DHFR protein with reduced affinity for MTX, have been observed in multiple cell lines following (in most cases) exposure to sequentially increased doses of the drug [81–84]. In order to determine if mutations in DHFR occur in patients, the blast samples from over twenty patients were tested for alterations in the binding of MTX to DHFR using an enzyme level MTX binding assay. The complete DHFR cDNA from blasts of eight patients, six ALL (four relapsed and two untreated) and two patients with untreated AML, were also analyses. While this represents only a small number of patient samples, we did not detect decreased MTX binding at the protein level, nor alterations in the coding region of the DHFR cDNA from any of these samples. In another study the cDNA for the DHFR gene was sequenced from seventeen patients with relapsed ALL who had been treated with MTX and no mutations were identified [85]. Thus, it seems unlikely that mutations in DHFR are a frequent mechanism of acquired resistance in patients exposed to MTX, although further studies may be warranted. It is of interest that the evolution of mutated DHFR in the organism *Plasmodium falciparum* has rendered the use of the DHFR inhibitor, pyrimethamine, ineffective as a malaria prophylactic in regions of the world where it saw widespread use [86].

Methotrexate resistance in osteosarcoma

Recently, MTX resistance was studied in osteosarcoma (OS). In this disease MTX administered at high doses with leucovorin rescue is a standard component of therapy, but when MTX is administered at conventional doses no responses are seen. It appears that a threshold serum MTX level is associated with improved patient chemotherapy response and outcome [87]. This is in contrast to the tumors described previously and it is unclear if this tumor should be considered intrinsically resistant or sensitive. RFC and DHFR mRNA expression were measured in tumors from 42 patients with OS using RT-PCR. 13 of the 20 (65%) OS samples were found to have decreased RFC expression at the time of initial biopsy [88]. Two of the 20 samples (10%) showed increased DHFR expression at initial biopsy. In metastatic or recurrent tumors the frequency of increased DHFR (62%, p=0.014) was significantly higher than at the time of initial biopsy whereas little change was observed in the frequency of decreased RFC expression [88]. The high frequency of decreased RFC expression in the biopsy material suggests impaired transport of methotrexate is a mechanism of intrinsic MTX resistance in OS. Increased DHFR expression in the pulmonary metastases may be a mechanism of acquired MTX resistance or a difference between primary and metastatic lesions [88].

Tumor suppressor genes and drug resistance

Loss of functional retinoblastoma protein (pRb) may also contribute to MTX resistance because cells lacking pRb may have increased levels of enzymes associated with proliferation as a consequence of increased levels of free E2F, a transcription factor that is sequestered by hypophosphorylated pRb. When cells transition from G1 into S phase, pRb becomes phosphorylated and releases the bound E2F which then enhances the transcription of genes involved in DNA synthesis, such as DHFR [89]. Increased DHFR protein levels lead to MTX resistance. The E2F-4 member of the E2F family of transcription factors has been most closely associated with the increase in DHFR transcription [90]. A human osteosarcoma cell line SaOS-2 that lacks pRb is intrinsically resistant to MTX as compared to lines with pRb present. This cell line has a higher level of DHFR and the increase in this activity is directly attributable to increased transcription of the DHFR gene. When the cDNA encoding pRb was reintroduced into this cell line sensitivity to MTX was restored. Other human sarcoma cell lines which lack pRb also show a similar level of resistance to MTX [91].

Since free or unbound E2F levels increase when pRb is hyperphosphorylated, activation of regulators of pRb phosphorylation, such as the cyclin dependent kinase system (cyclin D1-CDK4), may also cause an increase in DHFR transcription and hence MTX resistance. Transfection of cyclin D1 into the HT-1080 human sarcoma cell line resulted in an increase in MTX resistance in clones that expressed high levels of this gene, as compared to clones that expressed low levels, suggesting a direct relationship between the level of cyclin D1 expression and DHFR transcription [92]. Since certain tumors have been shown to express high levels of cyclin D1, MTX sensitivity may be decreased in these tumors. It is becoming increasingly clear that deregulation of cell cycle genes may have a profound effect on MTX resistance.

In cell lines with mutated p53, a tumor suppressor gene, amplification of genes occurs more readily [93, 94]. Mutations in the p53 gene were found in seven of the nine ALL blast samples associated with DHFR amplification. In contrast, only two of the 26 ALL blast samples without DHFR gene amplification had p53 mutations [79]. P53 mutations are therefore permissive for the development of MTX resistance through DHFR gene amplification. In this study, patients whose leukemic blasts demonstrated p53 mutations had a poor outcome [79].

New antifolates overcome methotrexate resistance

An understanding of the mechanisms underlying cellular resistance to MTX has directed the development of new therapeutic strategies which include the design of new agents and strategies where agents selectively target resistant cells. Several new antifolate inhibitors of DHFR and TS have been synthesized with attributes that may overcome or avoid the causes of intrinsic and acquired resistance to MTX (Fig. 3). That is, drugs that are either more efficiently converted to polyglutamate forms, may not require polyglutamylation for retention and efficacy, and/or do not require the RFC for cell entry [1].

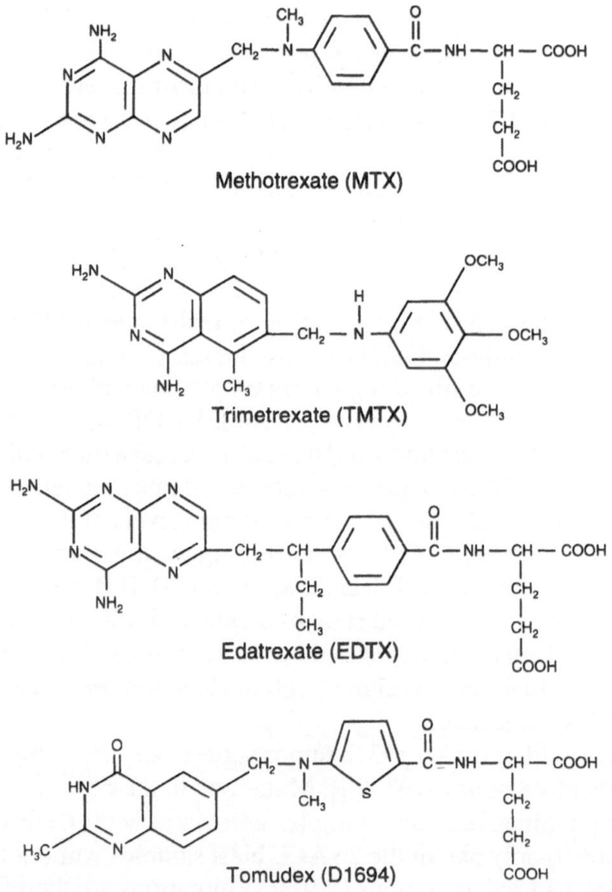

Figure 3. Chemical structures of newer antifolates.

Trimetrexate (TMTX), a lipophilic analog of MTX, has been studied extensively in recent years. It appears to have the advantage of not being dependent on the RFC for cell entry and, in some cells, is retained at high concentrations despite its inability to be polyglutamylated [95]. Recently, the finding that defective RFC transport is a common mechanism of MTX resistance in relapsed ALL and newly diagnosed OS has led to a heightened interest in this drug [74, 88]. Clinically, TMTX has had limited activity as a single agent in phase II clinical trials [96]. The major promise of TMTX may be in combination with other agents. The combination of TMTX and leucovorin (LV) is very active and non-toxic for the treatment of *Pneumocystis carinii* infections in acquired immunodeficiency syndrome (AIDS) patients [97]. The basis of this selectivity is that TMTX is transported by passive diffusion in this parasite, and LV can not rescue this organism because of its lack of RFC mediated transport. In combination, the side effects of TMTX on the host are eliminated since normal host cells are protected by LV [97]. This strategy has been applied to selectively target transport-defective tumors and similar results have been obtained *in vitro*. Severe combined immunodeficiency (SCID) mice bearing MTX resistant transport-defective ALL cells were tested with the combination of TMTX and LV, and marked tumor regression occurred without toxicity [98]. These studies have prompted a study using TMTX with LV protection (not rescue) in relapsed ALL and OS patients.

Edatrexate (EDTX), another MTX analog, is taken up and retained at higher concentrations than MTX in leukemic cells primarily due to its superior cellular import and better substrate activity for FPGS [96, 99]. However, as this drug also requires the RFC for cell entry and it also targets DHFR, some cross resistance to this drug in MTX resistant tumors may be expected [96, 100]. EDTX had promising activity as a single agent in phase II clinical trials. Response rates of 17 to 41% in breast cancer, 7 to 32% in non-small-cell lung cancer, 24 to 41% in head and neck cancer, 27% in non-Hodgkin's lymphoma and 14% in sarcomas (5 out of 7 with malignant fibrous histiocytoma responded) have been observed [96, 100, 101]. The toxicities of EDTX are similar to those observed with MTX, with mucositis and stomatitis being the dose limiting toxicities [96]. Phase III trials of EDTX in the treatment of sarcoma are anticipated in the near future.

Tomudex® (raltitrexed, D1694) is an antifolate inhibitor of the enzyme TS. Tomudex®, as compared to MTX, is a better substrate for the enzyme FPGS, and as a result is more efficiently polyglutamylated and retained [102]. In cell lines resistant to MTX on the basis of transport, cross-resistance with tomudex® is seen. Tomudex® has been tested in phase II clinical trials for a number of malignancies and particularly for colorectal carcinoma for which encouraging results were obtained (26% objective response rate) [102]. Phase III clinical trials in colorectal carcinoma comparing it to 5-fluorouracil treatment have demonstrated similar response rates with decreased costs and toxicity [103]. Tomudex® has been tested *in vitro* in leukemia cells and in AML it is more efficiently polyglutamylated and retained than is MTX. In addition it has an increased binding affinity for FPGS and may be worth testing in this disease [37].

Acknowledgement
I would like to acknowledge Dr. Joseph R Bertino for his guidance, support and encouragement. Richard Gorlick is supported by an American Society of Clinical Oncology Career Development Award.

References

1 Gorlick R, Goker E, Trippett T, Waltham M, Banerjee D, Bertino JR (1996) Intrinsic and acquired resistance to methotrexate in acute leukemia. *N Engl J Med* 335: 1041–1048
2 Farber S, Diamond LK, Mercer RD, Sylvester RF Jr, Wolff JA (1948) Temporary remissions in acute leukemia in children produced by folic acid antagonist, 4-aminopteroylglutamic acid (aminopterin). *N Engl J Med* 238: 787–793
3 Li MC, Hertz R, Spencer DB (1956) Effect of methotrexate therapy upon choriocarcinoma and chorioadenoma. *Proc Soc Exp Biol Med* 93: 361–366
4 Bertino JR (1993) Ode to methotrexate. *J Clin Oncol* 11: 5–14
5 Roberts RA, Nebert DW, Hickman JA, Richburg JH, Goldsworthy TL (1997) Perturbation of the mitosis/apoptosis balance: A fundamental mechanism in toxicology. *Fund Appl Toxicol* 38: 107–115
6 Chu E, Allegra CJ (1996) Antifolates. In: BA Chabner, DL Longo (eds): *Cancer Chemotherapy and Biotherapy*. Lippincott-Raven, Philadelphia, 109–148
7 Goldman ID, Lichenstein WS, Oliveiro VT (1968) Carrier-mediated transport of the folic acid analog methotrexate in the L1210 leukemia cell. *J Biol Chem* 243: 5007–5017
8 Sirotnak FM, Goutas LJ, Mines LS (1985) Extent of requirement for folate transport by L1210 cells for growth and leukemogenesis *in vivo*. *Cancer Res* 45: 4732–4734
9 Antony AC (1992) The biological chemistry of folate receptors. *Blood* 79: 2807–2820
10 Sierra EE, Brigle KE, Spinella MJ, Goldman ID (1997) pH dependence of methotrexate transport by the reduced folate carier and the folate receptor in L1210 leukemia cells – Further evidence for a third route mediated at a low pH. *Biochem Pharmacol* 53: 223–231
11 Assaraf YG, Babani S, Goldman ID (1998) Increased activity of a novel low pH folate transporter associated with lipophilic antifolate resistance in chinese hamster ovary cells. *J Biol Chem* 273: 8106–8111
12 Allegra CJ, Chabner BA, Drake JC, Lutz R, Rodbard D, Jolivet J (1985) Enhanced inhibition of thymidylate synthase by methotrexate polyglutamates. *J Biol Chem* 260: 9720–9726
13 Allegra CJ, Drake JC, Jolivet J, Chabner BA (1985) Inhibition of phosphoribosylaminoimidazole carboxamide transformylase by methotrexate and dihydrofolic acid polyglutamates. *Proc Natl Acad Sci USA* 82: 4881–4885
14 Anderson RG, Kamen BA, Rothberg KG, Lacey SW (1992) Potocytosis: sequestration and transport of small molecules by caveolae. *Science* 255: 410–411
15 Lacey SW, Sanders JM, Rothberg KG, Anderson RG, Kamen BA (1989) Complementary DNA for the folate binding protein correctly predicts anchoring to the membrane by glycosyl-phosphatidylinositol. *J Clin Invest* 84: 715–720
16 Spinella MJ, Brigle KE, Sierra EE, Goldman ID (1995) Distinguishing between folate receptor mediated transport and reduced folate carrier mediated transport in L1210 leukemia cells. *J Biol Chem* 270: 7842–7849
17 Williams FMR, Murray RC, Underhill TM, Flintoff WF (1994) Isolation of a hamster cDNA clone coding for a function involved in methotrexate uptake. *J Biol Chem* 269: 5810–5816
18 Dixon KH, Lampher BC, Chiu J, Kelley K, Cowan KH (1994) A novel cDNA restores reduced folate carrier activity and methotrexate sensitivity to transport deficient cells. *J Biol Chem* 269: 17–20

19 Williams FMR, Flintoff WF (1995) Isolation of a human cDNA that complements a mutant hamster cell defective in methotrexate uptake. *J Biol Chem* 270: 2987–2992

20 Moscow JA, Gong M, He R, Sgagias MK, Dixon KH, Anzick SL, Meltzer PS, Cowan KH (1995) Isolation of a gene encoding a human reduced folate carrier (RFC1) and analysis of its expression in transport-deficient methotrexate-resistant human breast cancer cells. *Cancer Res* 55: 3790–3795

21 Wong SC, Proefke SA, Bhushan A, Matherley LH (1995) Isolation of human cDNAs that restore methotrexate sensitivity and reduced folate carrier activity in methotrexate transport-defective Chinese hamster ovary cells. *J Biol Chem* 270: 17468–17475

22 Prasad PD, Ramamoorthy S, Leibach FH, Ganapathy V (1995) Molecular cloning of the human placental folate transporter. *Biochem Biophys Res Commun* 206: 681–687

23 Weitman SD, Lark RH, Coney LR, Fort DW, Frasca V, Zurawski VR, Kamen BA (1992) Distribution of the folate receptor GP38 in normal and malignant cell lines and tissues. *Cancer Res* 52: 3396–3401

24 Campbell IG, Jones TA, Foulkes WD, Trowsdale J (1991) Folate-binding protein is a marker for ovarian cancer. *Cancer Res* 51: 5329–5338

25 Westerhof GR, Rijnbout S, Schornagel JH, Pinedo HM, Peters GJ, Jansen G (1995) Functional activity of the reduced folate carrier in KB, MA104 and IGROV-1 cells expressing folate-binding protein. *Cancer Res* 55: 3795–3802

26 Sierra EE, Goldman ID (1998) Characterization of folate transport mediated by a low pH route in mouse L1210 leukemia cells with defective reduced folate carrier function. *Biochem Pharmacol* 55: 1505–1512

27 Assaraf YG, Goldman ID (1997) Loss of folic acid exporter function with markedly augmented folate accumulation in lipophilic antifolate-resistant mammalian cells. *J Biol Chem* 272: 17460–17466

28 Zhao R, Seither E, Brigle KE, Sharina IG, Wang PJ, Goldman ID (1997) Impact of over-expression of the reduced folate carrier (RFC1), an anion exchanger, on concentrative transport in murine L1210 leukemia cells. *J Biol Chem* 272: 21207–21212

29 Saxena M, Henderson GB (1996) MOAT4, a novel multi-specific organic-anion transporter for glucuronides and mercapturates in mouse L1210 cells and human erythrocytes. *Biochem J* 320: 273–281

30 Longo GSA, Gorlick R, Tong WP, Lin S, Steinherz P, Bertino JR (1997) Gamma-glutamyl hydrolase and folylpolyglutamate synthetase activities predict polyglutamylation of methotrexate in acute leukemias. *Oncol Res* 9: 259–263

31 Mcguire JJ, Hsieh P, Coward JK, Bertino JR (1980) Enzymatic synthesis of folylpolyglutamates. Characterization of the reaction and its products. *J Biol Chem* 255: 5776–5788

32 Garrow TA, Admon A, Shane B (1992) Expression cloning of a human cDNA encoding folylpoly (λ-glutamate) synthetase and determination of its primary structure. *Proc Natl Acad Sci USA* 89: 9151–9155

33 Chen L, Qi H, Korenberg J, Garrow TA, Choi YJ, Shane B (1996) Purification and properties of human cytosolic folylpoly-λ-glutamate synthetase and organization, localization, and differential splicing of its gene. *J Biol Chem* 271: 13077–13087

34 Roy K, Mitsugi K, Sirotnak FM (1996) Organization and alternate splicing of the murine folylpolyglutamate synthetase gene. *J Biol Chem* 271: 23820–23827

35 Roy K, Mitsugi K, Sirotnak FM (1997) Additional organizational features of the murine folylpolyglutamate synthetase gene. *J Biol Chem* 272: 5587-5593

36 Freemantle SJ, Moran RG (1997) Transcription of the human folyl-λ-glutamate synthetase gene. *J Biol Chem* 272: 25373–25379

37 Longo GSA, Gorlick R, Tong WP, Ercikan E, Bertino JR (1997) Disparate affinities of antifolates for folylpolyglutamate synthetase from human leukemia cells. *Blood* 90: 1241–1245

38 Galivan J, Johnson T, Rhee M, McGuire JJ, Priest D, Kesevan V (1987) The role of folylpolyglutamate synthesis and gamma-glutamyl hydrolase in altering cellular folyl- and anti-folylpolyglutamates. *Adv Enz Reg* 26: 147–155

39 Wang Y, Dias JA, Nimec Z, Rotundo RM, O'Connor BM, Freisheim J, Galivan J (1993) The properties and function of gamma-glutamyl hydrolase and poly-gamma-glutamate. *Adv Enz Reg* 33: 207–218

40 Samuels LL, Goutas LJ, Priest DG, Piper JR, Sirotnak FM (1986) Hydrolytic cleavage of methotrexate gamma-polyglutamates by folylpolyglutamyl hydrolase derived from various tumors and normal tissues of the mouse. *Cancer Res* 46: 2230–2235

41 Waltham MC, Li WW, Gritsman H, Tong WP, Bertino JR (1987) γ-Glutamyl hydrolase from human sarcoma HT-1080 cells: Characterization and inhibition by glutamine antagonists. *Molec Pharmacol* 51: 825–832

42 Yao R, Nimec Z, Ryan TJ, Galivan J (1996) Identification, cloning, and sequencing of a cDNA coding for rat γ-glutamyl hydrolase. *J Biol Chem* 271: 8525–8528

43 Yao R, Schneider E, Ryan TJ, Galivan J (1996) Human gamma-glutamyl hydrolase: cloning and characterization of the enzyme expressed *in vitro*. *Proc Natl Acad Sci USA* 93: 10134–10138

44 Bertino JR, Donohue DM, Simmons B, Gabrio BW, Silber R, Huennekens FM (1963) The induction of dihydrofolate reductase in leukocytes and erythrocytes of patients treated with methotrexate. *J Clin Invest* 42: 466–475

45 Chu E, Koeller DM, Casey JL, Drake JC, Chabner BA, Elwood PC, Zinn S, Allegra CA (1991) Autoregulation of human thymidylate synthase messenger RNA translation by thymidylate synthase. *Proc Natl Acad Sci USA* 88: 8977–8981

46 Hillcoat BL, Swett V, Bertino JR (1967) Increase of dihydrofolate reductase activity in cultured mammalian cells after exposure to methotrexate. *Proc Natl Acad Sci USA* 58: 1632–1637

47 Ercikan-Abali E, Banerjee D, Waltham MC, Skacel N, Scotto KW, Bertino JR (1997) Dihydrofolate reductase protein inhibits its own translation by binding to dihydrofolate reductase mRNA sequences within the coding region. *Biochemistry* 36: 12317–12322

48 Moscow JA, Connolly T, Myers TG, Cheng CC, Paull K, Cowan KH (1997) Reduced folate carrier gene (RFC1) expression and anti-folate resistance in transfected and non-selected cell lines. *Int J Cancer* 72: 184–190

49 Brigle KE, Spinella MJ, Sierra EE, Goldman ID (1995) Characterization of a mutation in the reduced folate carrier in a transport defective L1210 murine leukemia cell line. *J Biol Chem* 270: 22974–22979

50 Gong M, Yess J, Connolly T, Ivy SP, Ohnuma T, Cowan KH, Moscow JA (1997) Molecular mechanism of antifolate transport-deficiency in a methotrexate-resistant MOLT-3 human leukemia cell line. *Blood* 89: 2494–2499

51 Pizzorno G, Mini E, Coronnello M, McGuire JJ, Moroson BA, Cashmore AR, Dreyer RN, Lin JT, Mazzei T, Periti P et al (1988) Impaired polyglutamylation of methotrexate as a cause of resistance in CCRF-CEM cells after short-term, high-dose treatment with this drug. *Cancer Res* 48: 2149–2155

52 Tse A, Brigle K, Taylor SM, Moran RG (1998) Mutations in the reduced folate carrier gene which confer dominant resistance to 5,10-dideazatetrahydrofolate. *J Biol Chem* 273: 25953–25960

53 Pickard M, Kinsella A (1996) Influence of both salvage and DNA damage response pathways on resistance to chemotherapeutic antimetabolites. *Biochem Pharmacol* 52: 425–431

54 Wilson JK, Fischer PH, Remick SC, Tutsch KD, Grem JL, Nieting L, Alberti D, Bruggink J, Trump DL (1989) Methotrexate and dipyridamole combination chemotherapy based upon inhibition of nucleoside salvage in humans. *Cancer Res* 49: 1866–1870

55 Howell SB, Ensminger WD, Krishan A, Frei E (1978) Thymidine rescue of high-dose methotrexate in humans. *Cancer Res* 38: 325-330

56 Schweitzer BI, Dicker AP, Bertino JR (1990) Dihydrofolate reductase as a therapeutic target. *FASEB J* 4: 2441–2452

57 Li WW, Waltham M, Tong W, Schweitzer BI, Bertino JR (1993) Increased activity of gamma-glutamyl hydrolase in human sarcoma cell lines: a novel mechanism of intrinsic resistance to methotrexate. *Adv Exp Med Biol* 338: 635–638

58 Lin JT, Tong WP, Trippett TM, Niedzwiecki D, Tao Y, Tan C, Steinherz P, Schweitzer BI, Bertino JR (1991) Basis for natural resistance to methotrexate in human acute non-lymphocytic leukemia. *Leukemia Res* 15: 1191–1196

59 Goker E, Lin JT, Trippett T, Elisseyeff Y, Tong W, Niedzwiecki D, Tan C, Steinherz P, Schweitzer BI, Bertino JR (1993) Decreased polyglutamylation of methotrexate in acute lymphoblastic leukemia blasts in adults compared to children with this disease. *Leukemia* 7: 1000–1004

60 Goker E, Kheradpour A, Waltham M, Banerjee D, Tong WP, Elisseyeff Y, Bertino JR (1995) Acute monocytic leukemia: a myeloid subset that may be sensitive to methotrexate. *Leukemia* 9: 274–276

61 Hryniuk WM, Bertino JR (1969) Treatment of leukemia with large doses of methotrexate and folinic acid: clinical-biochemical correlates. *J Clin Invest* 48: 2140–2155

62 Rodenhuis S, Mcguire JJ, Narayanan R, Bertino JR (1986) Development of an assay system for the detection and classification of methotrexate resistance in fresh human leukemia cells. *Cancer Res* 46: 6513–6519

63 Li WW, Lin JT, Tong WP, Trippett TM, Brennan MF, Bertino JR (1992) Mechanisms of natural resistance to antifolates in human soft tissue sarcomas. *Cancer Res* 52: 1434–1438

64 Barakat RR, Li WW, Lovelace C, Bertino JR (1993) Intrinsic resistance of cervical cell carcinoma cell lines to methotrexate (MTX) as a result of decreased accumulation of intracellular MTX polyglutamates. *Gynecol Oncol* 93: 2255–2262

65 Pizzorno G, Chang YM, McGuire JJ, Bertino JR (1989) Inherent resistance of human squamous carcinoma cell lines to methotrexate as a result of decreased polyglutamylation of this drug. *Cancer Res* 49: 5275–5280

66 Barredo JC, Synold TW, Laver J, Relling MV, Pui CH, Priest DG, Evans WE (1994) Differences in constitutive and post-methotrexate folylpolyglutamate synthetase activity in B-lineage and T-lineage leukemia. *Blood* 84: 564–569

67 Synold TW, Relling MV, Boyett JM, Rivera GK, Sandlund JT, Mahmoud H, Crist WM, Pui CH, Evans WE (1994) Blast cell methotrexate-polyglutamate accumulation *in vivo* differs by lineage, ploidy, and methotrexate dose in acute lymphoblastic leukemia. *J Clin Invest* 94: 1996–2001

68 Whitehead VM, Rosenblatt DS, Vuchich MJ, Shuster JJ, Witte A, Beaulieu D (1990) Accumulation of methotrexate and methotrexate polyglutamates in lymphoblasts at diagnosis of childhood acute lymphoblastic leukemia: A pilot prognostic factor analysis. *Blood* 76: 44–49

69 Argiris A, Longo GSA, Gorlick R, Tong W, Steinherz P, Bertino JR (1997) Increased methotrexate polyglutamylation in acute megakaryocytic leukemia (M7) compared to other subtypes of acute myelocytic leukemia. *Leukemia* 11: 886–889

70 Galpin AJ, Schuetz JD, Masson E, Yanishevski Y, Synold TW, Barredo JC, Pui CH, Relling MV, Evans WE (1997) Differences in folylpolyglutamate synthetase and dihydrofolate reductase expression in human B-lineage vs. T-lineage leukemic lymphoblasts: Mechanisms for lineage differences in methotrexate polyglutamylation and cytotoxicity. *Molec Pharmacol* 52: 155–163

71 Rots MG, Pieters R, Noordhuis P, Van Zantwijk CH, Peters GJ, Veerman AJP, Jansen G (1997) Role of folylpolyglutamate synthetase (FPGS) and folylpolyglutamate hydrolase (FPGH) in methotrexate (MTX) polyglutamylation in childhood leukemia. *Proc Amer Accos Cancer Res* 33: A1088

72 Lenz HJ, Danenberg K, Schnieders B, Goker E, Peters GJ, Garrow T, Shane B, Bertino JR, Danenberg PV (1994) Quantitative analysis of folylpolyglutamate synthetase gene expression in tumor tissues by the polymerase chain reaction: Marked variation of expression among leukemia patients. *Oncol Res* 6: 329–335

73 Trippett T, Schlemmer S, Elisseyeff Y, Goker E, Wachter M, Steinherz P, Tan C, Berman E, Wright JE, Rosowsky A (1992) Defective transport as a mechanism of acquired resistance to methotrexate in patients with acute leukemia. *Blood* 80: 1158–1162

74 Gorlick R, Goker E, Trippett T, Steinherz P, Elisseyeff Y, Mazumdar M, Flintoff WF, Bertino JR (1997) Defective transport is a common mechanism of acquired methotrexate resistance in acute lymphocytic leukemia and is associated with decreased reduced folate carrier expression. *Blood* 89: 1013–1018

75 Zhang L, Taub JW, Williamson M, Wong SC, Hukku B, Pullen J, Ravindranath Y, Matherley LH (1998) Reduced folate carrier expression in childhood acute lymphoblastic leukemia: Relationship to immunophenotype and ploidy. *Clin Cancer Res* 4: 2169–2177

76 Schimke RT (1988) Gene amplification in cultured cells. *J Biol Chem* 263: 5989–5992

77 Srimatkandada S, Medina WD, Cashmore AR, Whyte W, Engel D, Moroson BA, Franco CT, Dube SK, Bertino JR (1983) Amplification and organization of dihydrofolate reductase genes in a human leukemia cell line, K-562, resistant to methotrexate. *Biochemistry* 22: 5774–5781

78 Stark GR, Debatisse M, Guilotto E, Wahl GM (1989) Recent progress in understanding mechanisms of mammalian DNA amplification. *Cell* 57: 901–908
79 Goker E, Waltham M, Kheradpour A, Trippett T, Mazumdar M, Elisseyeff Y, Schnieders B, Steinherz P, Tan C, Berman E et al (1995) Amplification of the dihydrofolate reductase gene is a mechanism of acquired resistance to methotrexate in patients with acute lymphocytic leukemia and is correlated with p53 gene mutations. *Blood* 86: 677–684
80 Matherly LH, Taub JW, Wong SC, Simpson PM, Ekizian R, Buck S, Williamson M, Amylon M, Pullen J, Camitta B et al (1997) Increased frequency of expression of elevated dihydrofolate reductase in T-cell vs. B-precursor acute lymphoblastic leukemia in children. *Blood* 90: 578–589
81 Haber DA, Beverly SM, Kiely ML, Schimke RT (1981) Properties of an altered dihydrofolate reductase encoded by amplified genes in cultured mouse fibroblasts. *J Biol Chem* 256: 9501–9510
82 Srimatkandada S, Schweitzer BI, Moroson BA, Dube S, Bertino JR (1989) Amplification of a polymorphic dihydrofolate reductase gene expressing an enzyme with a decreased binding to Methotrexate in a human colon carcinoma cell line, HCT-8R4, resistant to this drug. *J Biol Chem* 264: 3524–3528
83 Melera PW, Davide JP, Hession CA, Scotto KW (1984) Phenotypic expression in Escherichia coli and nucleotide sequence of two Chinese hamster lung cDNAs encoding different dihydrofolate reductases. *Mol Cell Biol* 4: 38–48
84 Dicker AP, Volkenandt M, Schweitzer BI, Banerjee D, Bertino JR (1990) Identification and characterization of a mutation in the dihydrofolate reductase gene from methotrexate-resistant Chinese hamster ovary cell line Pro-3 Methotrexate RIII. *J Biol Chem* 265: 8317–8321
85 Spencer HT, Sorrentino BP, Pui CH, Chunduru SK, Sleep SEH, Blakley RL (1996) Mutations in the gene for human dihydrofolate reductase: an unlikely cause of clinical relapse in pediatric leukemia patients after therapy with methotrexate. *Leukemia* 10: 439–446
86 Hyde JE (1990) The dihydrofolate reductase-thymidylate synthetase gene in the drug resistance of malaria parasites. *Pharmacol Therapeutics* 48: 45–59
87 Bacci G, Ferrari S, Delepine N, Bertoni F, Picci P, Mercuri M, Bacchini P, Brach del Prever A, Tienghi A, Comandone A et al (1998) Predictive factors of histologic response to primary chemotherapy in osteosarcoma of the extremity: study of 272 patients preoperatively treated with high-dose methotrexate, doxorubicin, and cisplatin. *J Clin Oncol* 16: 658–663
88 Guo W, Healey JH, Meyers PA, Ladanyi M, Huvos AG, Bertino JR, Gorlick R (1999) Mechanisms of methotrexate resistance in osteosarcoma. *Clin Cancer Res* 5: 621–627
89 Nevins JR (1992) E2F a link between the Rb tumor suppressor protein and viral oncoproteins. *Science* 258: 424–429
90 Wells JM, Illenye S, Magae J, Wu, CL, Heintz NH (1997) Accumulation of E2F-4-DP-1 DNA binding complexes correlates with induction of dhfr gene expression during the G_1 to S phase transition. *J Biol Chem* 272: 4483–4492
91 Li WW, Fan J, Hochhauser D, Banerjee D, Zielenski Z, Almasan A, Yin Y, Kelly R, Wahl GM, Bertino JR (1995) Absence of functional retinoblastoma protein mediates increased resistance to antimetabolites in human sarcoma cell lines. *Proc Natl Acad Sci USA* 92: 10436–10440
92 Hochhauser D, Schnieders B, Ercikan-Abali E, Gorlick R, Muise-Helmericks R, Li WW, Fan J, Banerjee D, Bertino JR (1996) Effect of cyclin D1 overexpression on drug sensitivity in a human fibrosarcoma cell line. *J Natl Cancer Inst* 88: 1269–1275
93 Livingstone LR, White A, Sprouse J, Livanos E, Jacks T, Tlsty TD (1992) Altered cell cycle arrest and gene amplification potential accompany loss of wild-type p53. *Cell* 70: 923–935
94 Yin Y, Tainsky MA, Bischoff FZ, Strong LC, Wahl GM (1992) Wild-type p53 restores cell cycle control and inhibits gene amplification in cells with mutant p53 alleles. *Cell* 70: 937–948
95 Kamen BA, Eibl B, Cashmore A, Bertino JR (1984) Uptake and efficacy of trimetrexate (TMQ, 2,2-diamino-5-methyl-6-[(3,4,5-trimethoxyanilino)methyl] quinazoline), a nonclassical antifolate in methotrexate-resistant leukemia cells *in vitro*. *Biochem Pharmacol* 33: 1697–1699

96 Takimoto CH, Allegra CJ (1995) New antifolates in clinical development. *Oncol* 9: 649–656

97 Allegra CJ, Chabner BA, Tuazon CU, Ogata-Arakaki D, Baird B, Drake JC, Simmons JT, Lack EE, Shelhamer JH, Balis F (1987) Trimetrexate for the treatment of pneumocystis carinii pneumonia in patients with the acquired immunodeficiency syndrome. *N Engl J Med* 317: 978–985

98 Lacerda JF, Goker E, Kheradpour A, Dennig D, Elisseyeff Y, Jagiello C, O'Reilly RJ, Bertino JR (1995) Selective treatment of SCID mice bearing methotrexate-transport-resistant human acute lymphoblastic leukemia tumors with trimetrexate and leucovorin protection. *Blood* 85: 2675–2679

99 Sirotnak FM, Schmid FA, Samuels LL, Degraw JI (1987) 10-Ethyl-10-deaza-aminopterin: structural design and biochemical, pharmacological, and antitumor properties. *Natl Cancer Inst Monographs* 5: 127-131

100 Grant SC, Kris MG, Young CW, Sirotnak FM (1993) Edatrexate: an antifolate with antitumor activity: a review. *Cancer Invest* 11: 36–45

101 Casper ES, Christman KL, Schwartz GK, Johnson B, Brennan MF, Bertino JR (1993) Edatrexate in patients with soft tissue sarcoma. Activity in malignant fibrous histiocytoma. *Cancer* 72: 766–770

102 Takemura Y, Jackman AL (1997) Folate-Based thymidylate synthase inhibitors in cancer chemotherapy. *Anti-Cancer Drugs* 8: 3–16

103 Cunningham D (1998) Mature results from three large controlled studies with raltitrexed ('Tomudex'). *Br J Cancer* 77: 15–21

Methotrexate
ed. by B. N. Cronstein und J. R. Bertino
© 2000 Birkhäuser Verlag Basel/Switzerland

Current use of methotrexate in the treatment of malignancies in adults

James O'Leary, Alexander Losev and Franco M. Muggia

Kaplan Comprehensive Cancer Center, NYU Medical Center, 550 First Avenue, New York, NY 10016, USA

Introduction

This chapter reviews major indications for the use of methotrexate in the treatment of adult malignancies. These indications have evolved in relation to the introduction of new therapeutic modalities. However, the prominent role played by methotrexate in the past continues to be assessed and may be expected to be reconsidered within our therapeutic armamentarium. For this reason we have given added focus to pharmacological principles, and the use of high dose methotrexate.

Uses of methotrexate

Gestational trophoblastic disease

In 1956, the introduction of methotrexate (MTX) to treat gestational trophoblastic disease (GTD) revolutionized the treatment and outcome of this disease. For non-metastatic GTD, the cure rate reached almost 100%. Prior to the introduction of chemotherapy, surgery with hysterectomy achieved a five-year survival of only 41%. As such, surgery began to play a diminished role and was subsequently used only for initial evacuation of the mole. Hammond, Hertz, and Li reported the marked efficacy of single-agent MTX in treating non-metastatic GTD and it was rapidly incorporated into clinical practice. When given at a dose of 15 to 25 mg intramuscularly (IM) every day for five days, 93% of those treated achieved a complete remission (CR). However, there was substantial toxicity associated with this regimen: alopecia, neutropenia, and mucositis. In an attempt to reduce toxicity, Berkowitz and Goldstein administered the MTX at a dose of 1 mg/kg IM every other day for four doses with leucovorin at a dose of 0.1 mg/kg IM 24 hours after each dose of MTX. With this newer regimen, 90% of those treated achieved a sustained remission while toxicity was markedly reduced. 87% of the patients showed a 10-fold decrease in their human chorionic gonadotrophin (hCG) level after only one cycle of chemotherapy. These patients were able to maintain a remission without any further therapy. Hence, the Berkowitz-Goldstein regimen was widely adopted for non-metastatic GTD. Next, the Gynecologic Oncology Group (GOG) investigated the possibility of utilizing weekly single-agent MTX at a dose of 30 to 50 mg/m². Patients were treated until hCG levels had normalized for three consecutive weeks. This cost-effective and well-tolerated regimen replaced the Berkowitz and Goldstein regimen as the standard of care for treating non-metastatic GTD. The GOG also investigated the activity of Actinomycin-D at a dose of 1.25 mg/m² intravenously every two weeks. They concluded that Actinomycin-D given in this fashion was as effective as MTX given on a weekly schedule. Both regimens were safe, inexpensive, effective, and a convenient therapy. Actinomycin-D has more vesicant and emetogenic potential. Hence, MTX continues to be the drug of choice for the first line treatment of GTD [1–5] that is low risk. This definition includes both sites of disease and the hCG level, and requires computerized tomography to ensure no metastases beyond pelvis or lung.

Patients with high risk GTD require combination chemotherapy. High risk GTD patients are those that present with disease greater than four months after an antecedent pregnancy, those with a pretreatment hCG level greater than 100,000 IU/24 hour urine or greater than 40,000 mIU/ml serum, those with metastases to sites other than lung or vagina, those with antecedent term gestation, and those who have failed prior therapy [6, 7]. These patients are not likely to be cured by single-agent chemotherapy. The benefit of combination therapy for this group of patients was first noted in 1968. Patients treated with the MAC regimen, (MTX, Actinomycin, and cyclophosphamide) had a survival rate of 65% compared to 39% in patients who were treated with single-agent therapy followed by MAC. The MAC regimen was standard care throughout the 1970s [6].

In the early 1980s, etoposide was found to be very active and the EMA/CO regimen (alternating etoposide, high dose MTX, and Actinomycin-D with cyclophosphamide and vincristine) was formulated by Newlands and it replaced the prior MAC regimen. MTX is administered as 100 mg intravenous (IV) bolus followed by 200 mg continuous IV infusion over 12 hours. Treatment with EMA/CO is well tolerated with little severe toxicity, achieves high response rates, and good long-term survival rates. This favorable profile makes the EMA/CO the initial treatment of choice for high-risk patients [5, 6]. The regimen has resulted in cure rates of 80–90% in patients with high risk GTD [5]. Colony-stimulating factors should be used when needed in order to avoid treatment delays [6, 8]. This intensive chemotherapy has a small risk of inducing secondary malignancies (acute myeloid leukemia, cervical cancer, and gastric adenocarcinoma) reported by Newland in an analysis of 272 consecutive patients treated at Charing Cross Hospital between 1979 and 1995. The development of secondary leukemias argues for limiting etoposide exposure to patients at highest risk [5, 9–12]. On the other hand, patients at high risk may be best treated by a platinum-based regimen, including etoposide, but avoiding the alkylating agents.

Bladder cancer

Urothelial cancers are now recognized to be chemotherapeutically responsive tumors. The incidence of bladder cancer has increased by 36% over the last ten years. During the same time interval, there has been 8% improvement in survival rates [13, 14] Chemotherapy has made a substantial impact on the treatment of bladder cancer. From pooled phase II data, single-agent cisplatin therapy has a response rate of 30% while MTX shows a response rate of 29% [15]. MTX has been studied extensively using various modes and schedules of administration and an overall response rate of 36% was noted at doses of 50 mg, 100 mg, or 200 mg IV with leucovorin rescue. Combination regimens that contain both agents have consistently produced high response rates, a number of complete responses, as well as prolonged duration of response. The most commonly used standard chemotherapy regimens are MVAC (MTX, vinblastine, doxorubicin, and cisplatin) and CMV (cisplatin, MTX, and vincristine). Overall response rates to combination regimens range from 50 to 70%, with complete responses seen in 10 to 20%. The median survival is approximately one year [13–19]. In a large intergroup study, MVAC was compared to single-agent cisplatin and a progression-free and overall survival advantage was shown for those patients treated with the combination regimen [16]. The study also identified several poor risk prognosticators which included poor performance status, bone or visceral involvement, and non-transitional-cell histology [16–17].

For metastatic disease, therefore, combination chemotherapy with MVAC is the current standard with an overall response rate (RR) of 35% to 45% and a median survival of 12 months [15, 16, 20]. The regimen was originally described by Sternberg from the Memorial Sloan-Kettering Cancer Center. In a trial at the M. D. Anderson Cancer Center, MVAC was compared to CISCA (cisplatin, cyclophosphamide, and doxorubicin). MVAC showed a superior response rate of 65% compared to 46% seen with CISCA and a modest advantage in survival [21]. The overall RR for MVAC in phase III trials is about 50%, but the overall cure rate is low [14]. Escalated doses of MVAC with granulocyte colony-stimulating factor support increases the response rate but not overall survival [14, 15].

A number of trials have evaluated the effectiveness of neoadjuvant therapy for patients with invasive disease. The goals of neoadjuvant treatment are to control micrometastases more effectively and improve overall survival, while treating local disease and allowing organ preservation. Such treatment also helps to determine the sensitivity of the tumor to initial chemotherapy allowing subsequent alteration of therapy as needed. In one study using MVAC, the number of tumors that could be removed by partial cystectomy as opposed to complete cystectomy increased by 27% [22]. In a large intercontinental study, (MRC/EORTC Trial) 975 patients with muscle invasive bladder cancer were randomized to four arms: CMV X 3 followed by radical cystectomy, radical cystectomy alone, full-dose external beam radiotherapy, or preoperative radiation followed by cystectomy. Although no difference in overall survival have been detected so far, 33% of patients who were treated neoadjuvantly did not have a tumor in the cystectomy specimen compared to 12% of patients who were not treated preoperatively [23].

More recently, other drugs such as gemcitabine and paclitaxel have been introduced and combinations often exclude methotrexate. An exception is a proposed salvage regimen consisting of MTX, paclitaxel, and cisplatin. Partial responses were seen in ten of 25 patients with refractory disease with three of the responses remarkably occurring in seven patients with liver metastases [13, 24].

Gastric carcinoma

Adenocarcinoma of the stomach is one of the leading causes of cancer death worldwide and still one of the most common types of cancers in the United States. Most patients present either with unresectable disease, or promptly relapse leading to a 5–15% 5-year survival rate. Systemic chemotherapy has had an uncertain impact on survival. In the late 1980's Klein and co-workers popularized sequential high dose methotrexate followed by 5-FU (5-fluorouracil), in combination with doxorubicin (FAMTX) for advanced gastric cancer. These investigators observed a 63% response rate but survival was not obviously better than in prior studies [25]. The rationale for MTX-5FU sequences was initially provided by Bertino and co-workers – see chapter I. The therapeutic effect of 5-FU can be potentiated by the methotrexate-induced increase in the pool of phosphoribosylpyrophosphate (PRPP) resulting in increased 5-FU ribonucleotide metabolites. In turn, PRPP availability also increases incorporation of those fluorinated metabolites into RNA.

In the early 1990's several phase III studies were reported in which best supportive care was compared to this systemic chemotherapy. Those regimens studied showed a modest prolongation of survival with chemotherapy. In some studies up to 40% of patients were alive at one year but only 10% at two years [26–29]. Proving that chemotherapy was better than palliative care paved the way for comparison of different chemotherapeutic regimens. In the study of FAMTX vs. EAP (Etoposide, Doxorubicin, Cisplatin) FAMTX proved to be as active as EAP but with significantly less toxicity [27]. A prospective phase III multicenter trial of FAMTX vs. FAM

(5-FU, Doxorubicin, Mitomycin) showed a significantly superior response rate (41% vs. 9%, p < 0.0001) and survival (median, 42 weeks vs. 29 weeks, p = 0.004) of FAMTX over FAM [28]. Toxicity was manageable and comparable in both regimens. Subsequently, in a trial which compared FAMTX vs. ECF (Epirubicin, Cisplatin, 5-FU) [29], FAMTX was shown to be inferior in terms of response rate (45% with ECF and 21% with FAMTX, p = 0.0002) and median survival (8.9 months with ECF and 5.7 months with FAMTX, p = 0.0009). At one year 36% of ECF patients and 21% of FAMTX patients were alive. In that study, the FAMTX regimen caused more hematological toxicity and serious infections while ECF caused more emesis and alopecia. Thus, variable advantages for any one regimen mitigate against considering any one of these regimens as a standard. More recently, the use of 5-FU-based neoadjuvant therapies and topoisomerase-1 inhibitors have given rise to new regimens that may be more effective and are therefore replacing FAMTX.

Head and neck cancers

The median survival for patients with local or disseminated recurrent squamous cell carcinoma of the head and neck is six months. Only about 20% of patients survive at one-year [30]. Chemotherapy with single-agents like methotrexate, bleomycin, cisplatin, 5-FU, taxanes, or with combinations like 5-FU and cisplatin failed to make any significant impact on survival in these patients, and are used mostly as a palliative therapy. More intense regiments like 5-FU and cisplatin or the single-agents taxol or taxetere are limited to patients with good performance status who are able to tolerate the toxicities of these regimens. Methotrexate is a well-established and well-tolerated drug in this patient population. It is usually initiated at 40 mg/m^2 weekly. Several randomized trials [30–32] failed to show any superiority of high dose methotrexate, with leucovorin rescue, over conventional dose methotrexate (Tab. 1). Current regimens have not included methotrexate in the neoadjuvant or advanced disease treatment, since a comparative study by the Southwest Oncology Group showed cisplatin + 5FU to be superior in response rate [33].

Primary central nervous system lymphoma (PCNSL)

Primary central nervous system lymphoma is an aggressive non-Hodgkin's lymphoma that arises within the brain, spinal cord, leptomeninges, or eye. It represents 5% of all brain tumors. Most patients with PCNSL are immunocompetent. However, patients with acquired and congenital immunodeficiencies are at significantly greater risk for the development of this malignancy. Until relatively recently, treatment consisted of cranial

Table 1

Author	No. of patients	Methotrexate regimen	Response rate	Survival
Taylor et al. [31]	47	MTX 1.5 g/m^2 + leucovorin every week vs. 40 mg/m^2 every week	32% vs. 22%	4.2 months vs. 4.2 months
DeConti and Schoenfeld [32]	259	MTX 40–60 mg/m^2 every week vs. MTX 240 mg/m^2 + leucovorin every two weeks vs. MTX 240 mg + leucovorin + cytosine arobinoside + cyclophosphamide every two weeks	26% vs. 24% vs. 18%	186 days vs. 129 days vs. 81 days
Woods et al. [30]	58	MTX 5 g/m^2 weekly vs. 500 mg/m^2 weekly vs. 50 mg/m^2 weekly	50% vs. 21% vs. 31%	no survival difference

radiation therapy and corticosteroids. Historically, it produced a five-year survival rate of only 5-10%. With the recognition that radiation therapy alone is not curative for primary central nervous system lymphoma and the successful use of chemotherapy in systemic lymphomas, major emphasis has been shifted to adding systemic therapy.

PCNSL presents several unique challenges to the effective use of chemotherapy. One challenge may be related to the underrepresentation of immunological effector cells which may modulate the antitumor effect of chemotherapy within the CNS. Another challenge, often mentioned, is that of ensuring adequate delivery of the drugs to the brain parenchyma, or overcoming the so-called 'blood brain barrier'. The blood brain barrier results from the unique vascular bed of the brain, as compared to other vascular beds, which contains tight junctions between vascular endothelial cells compared to the fenestrations found between the endothelial cells in most other parts of the body. These junctions effectively eliminate any passive diffusion of large water-soluble molecules from the blood to the CNS. There is evidence that these cells actively pump out toxic substances. Nitrosoureas are capable of penetrating the blood brain barrier because of their lipid-soluble properties. In conventional doses methotrexate does not penetrate the blood brain barrier well. However, this is overcome by use of high dose regimens with leucovorin rescue. Some have disputed the relevance of such a barrier to chemotherapeutic regimens because the vascular bed in tumor-bearing areas may differ from that in the rest of the CNS.

The addition of methotrexate-based chemotherapy to cranial radiation therapy has improved both disease-free and overall survival. Some studies reported only a short follow up, but some showed median survival of over 30 months [34–41]. A recent follow-up study of methotrexate, cranial radiation therapy and high dose cytarabine conducted at the Memorial Sloan Kettering Cancer Center [41] reported a median survival of 42 months, with a five year survival of 22%. Results were significantly better than historical controls. These results also support using chemotherapy alone in patients above 60 years of age, since cranial radiation causes encephalopathy and this is aggravated when combined with methotrexate [42–44]. Of the patients enrolled in the study which combined chemotherapy and radiation, nearly 80% of one-year survivors over the age of 60 developed progressive encephalopathy. In younger populations, administering methotrexate before radiation therapy may diminish the risk of encephalopathy. Optimal management of primary central nervous system lymphoma is still evolving since most chemotherapy regimens and the timing or need for radiation therapy have yet to be determined.

Treatment of immunocompromised patients with PCNSL (AIDS patients being the largest group) has not been as successful and is generally considered palliative. In this group of patients PCNSL appears most often towards the terminal stages of their underlying disease when the CD4 counts are below 100 cells/dl. Most of these patients have a poor performance status, which limits their tolerance of chemotherapy. Their prognosis is extremely poor with most dying within 2–5 months from systemic or CNS infections. Chemotherapy treatment is usually limited to patients with a good performance status, no active comorbid conditions, and a CD4 cell count >200 [45]. These patients have benefited from regimens containing methotrexate. All other patients with AIDS should probably receive only palliative radiation therapy to the cranium, and corticosteroids.

Adult acute lymphoblastic leukemia (ALL)

ALL is currently subdivided into three classes. The most common subtype of ALL is pre-B cell. Cells in this subtype are committed to the B cell lineage, but they do not express the hallmark of mature B cells, surface immunoglobulins. This subtype of ALL represents approximately 70% of adult patients. The second subtype is T-cell lymphoblastic lymphoma/leukemia. It most often presents as a rapidly growing mediastinal mass with frequent involvement of the bone marrow early in the process. This subtype represents about 25% of adult ALL cases. Therapy is usually the same as for the pre-B cell subtype. The third subtype of adult ALL is mature B-cell ALL. It is called mature because it expresses surface IgG. It is the least common subtype and occurs in only about 5% of adult ALL. It is usually a disease of young adults who present with a rapidly growing abdominal mass and symptoms of pain, bloating, and small bowel obstruction. Bone marrow and CNS involvement occur very often. Treatment of mature B-cell ALL is very much different from the other two types of ALL.

The outcome of adults with ALL is worse than in the pediatric population. The poorer prognosis is in part attributed to the decreased ability of adults to tolerate intense chemotherapy coupled with an incidence of unfavorable cytogenetics e.g. Philadelphia chromosome positive ALL. Nevertheless, because of the high success rate that has been achieved in the pediatric population treatment of adults with ALL has been modeled on therapy developed for pediatric ALL. Treatment of ALL is generally divided into four categories: induction, consolidation, maintenance, and CNS prophylaxis. Induction typically consists of four or five chemotherapy drugs consisting of anthracyclines, cyclophosphamide, asparaginase, vincristine, and prednisone. Intensive consolidation therapy is based on cytarabine combined with anthracyclines, epidophyllotoxins, or methotrexate. The two-year maintenance therapy is based on oral methotrexate combined with 6-mercaptopurine. An integral part of the treatment is also prophylactic intrathecal chemotherapy with methotrexate. Patients who do not have CNS prophylaxis have a cumulative risk of approximately 35% of developing CNS involvement during the course of their disease.

As mentioned above, methotrexate plays an important role in L1 and L2 subtypes of ALL. It is even more important in the treatment regimen for L3 or what is often called small non-cleaved cell or Burkitt's lymphoma. Again, regimens that showed very encouraging results in pediatric Burkitt's lymphoma tend to be used for adults. The study published by Magrath et al. [46] reported event free survival of 92% at two years and beyond (no events occurred after two years). Even in patients with heavy bone marrow involvement, event-free survival was 80%. High risk patients (more than one site of involvement, high lactic dehydrogenase (LDH) received only four cycles of chemotherapy given over a period of 15 weeks regardless of the extent of disease. A key principle in therapy is rapid cycling of drugs (cyclophosphamide, methotrexate, cytarabine, doxorubicin, etoposide). Tumor lysis has been described in these situations and requires caution when methotrexate is used, because of a possible delay in renal excretion causing marked aggravation in toxicity. Methotrexate in this regimen is given as a high dose. Again, an intensive CNS prophylaxis, usually with methotrexate, is an integral part of the treatment. Similar results were reported by the French Pediatric Oncology Society using the same drugs on a different schedule [47].

Osteosarcoma

Prior to the 1970s, amputation and surgical resection was the mainstay of treatment for osteosarcoma of the extremities, a malignancy of adolescents and young adults. With this mode of therapy the overall survival for patients was about 20%. The majority of patients recurred in the lungs at six to nine months after amputation. This pattern of recurrence suggested that micrometastatic disease existed at the time of surgery. The original premise that osteosarcoma was a chemoresistant tumor was disproved by studies conducted in the 1970s which demonstrated that it was sensitive to three chemotherapeutic agents: high dose methotrexate (MTX), doxorubicin, and cisplatin [48]. Favorable results were observed in disease-free survival in patients treated with these agents vs. historical control patients treated with surgery alone (40% vs. 20% in five years) provided the impetus to attempt limb-sparing operative procedures [49]. With more modern approaches, chemotherapy has an even more significant impact in increasing disease-free survival, in the range of 65 to 75%. The benefit of adjuvant therapy is probably a result of controlling micrometastatic pulmonary disease, and such benefits have become even more apparent with the advent of preoperative (neoadjuvant) chemotherapy [48, 50].

Significant predictive factors for disease-free survival have been identified for patients with classical osteosarcoma localized to the extremity without any evidence of clinically detectable metastases. These include: chemotherapy-induced tumor necrosis in the primary tumor, baseline LDH serum value, and use of high dose MTX [51]. Maximal dose intensification of doxorubicin and MTX have been considered as important determinants of outcome [52]. In one institutional experience, in a multivariate analysis, the dose intensity of MTX was the most important factor in predicting outcome in non-metastatic osteosarcoma [51, 53, 54]. Others have found that cisplatin dose-intensity, but not MTX, improved results. In one study, the MTX dose was pharmacokinetically monitored and adapted to achieve the highest area under the concentration-time curve. The patients treated in this manner showed higher histological response rates and higher overall five-year survival. The investigators contend that the dose of MTX is such an important determinant of outcome that high dose MTX treatment should be adapted to individual pharmacokinetics [55]; however, these concepts require independent prospective confirmation.

These pharmacological correlates of response to MTX have shown that in patients with localized disease, the most important factors that influence necrosis are histology and the peak serum level of MTX. The highest degree of tumor necrosis was seen in telangiectatic and fibroblastic tumors. The lowest response was seen in chondroblastic tumors. The peak serum level of MTX significantly influences tumor necrosis. It is recommended that the serum level of MTX should be greater than 700 micromol/l [56].

Significantly higher serum mean peaks were observed in patients with complete tumor necrosis:

Peak MTX level (micromol/l)	Percentage necrosis
773.8	100%
649.1	90–99%
639.8	50–89%
610.0	less than 50%

MTX peak levels greater than 800 umol/l were not associated with a further increase in the amount of tumor necrosis [57]. When MTX infusion is prolonged, a dose adaptation is recommended to maintain the serum peak at a level greater than or equal to 770 µmol/l [56].

Due to the controversial results with the use of high dose MTX in single institution studies, a large multi-variate analysis was conducted. Through a computerized literature search, all published clinical trials of high dose MTX from 30 institutions comprising 1909 patients were analyzed. Whether given adjuvantly or neoadjuvantly, in combination therapy or as a single agent therapy, MTX dose intensity was a major factor in predicting outcome. No other drug or drug dose intensity correlated with disease-free survival as significantly as MTX [54]. These results may also reflect the use of high doses of MTX confined to younger patients and at certain institutions, resulting in better outcome.

Although the superiority of neoadjuvant chemotherapy compared to adjuvant chemotherapy still needs to be proved [49, 58], primary chemotherapy has emerged as the standard of care [59]. Preoperative chemotherapy has facilitated surgical resection of the primary bone tumor, making more patients candidates for limb-sparing surgery [48]. The percentage of amputations for osteosarcoma of the extremity has decreased by 80% [50]. Also, the effects of primary chemotherapy on the tumor is now used as a predictive factor for determining outcome. Many investigators have reported on the strong correlation between chemotherapy-induced necrosis and prognosis. The major benefit of preoperative chemotherapy is the ability to analyze which patients respond to the initial regimen and then to modify the postoperative regimen accordingly [48, 49, 59]. If the extent of necrosis in the primary tumor exceeded 90%, the chance for survival exceeded 80% [48]. Therefore, patients who are found to have a good response, as judged by the percent of necrosis to these drugs given neoadjuvantly, are continued on the same two drugs postoperatively. In poor responders, treatment is intensified by adding ifosfamide and other drugs to the regimens.

In a recent study, 55 patients with high-grade osteosarcoma were treated with neoadjuvant ifosfamide, doxorubicin and high dose MTX. Patients with a poor histological response had cisplatin added to the regimen post-operatively. For patients with tumor necrosis greater than or equal to 95%, the relapse – free survival and overall survival at six years were 79% and 88% respectively. If tumor necrosis was less than 95%, six year relapse free survival was 58% and overall survival was 83% [60].

Future directions in the treatment of osteosarcoma may include the use of targeted delivery of MTX to the bone tumor, using a MTX-bisphospho-nate conjugate. In experimental animal models, the conjugate was found to have five times the antineoplastic activity of MTX used alone [61]. Another possibility in improving the outcome of therapy is to test for genetic alterations before instituting therapy. Increased p21 expression has been found to correlate with increased sensitivity to MTX in cell lines [62].

Leptomeningeal cancer

About 8% of patients with cancer develop diffuse infiltration of the lepto-meninges. The cranial and spinal nerve roots are usually affected. The most common tumors that involve leptomeninges include non-Hodgkin's lymphoma, leukemia, melanoma, and adenocarcinomas of breast and lung origins. Traditionally, the treatment of meningeal carcinomatosis involves intrathecal chemotherapy and/or radiation. Chemotherapy is given either through the lumbar puncture into or preferably via an Ommaya type reservoir connected to a lateral ventricle. Most common chemotherapy agents include methotrexate, cytarabine (since 1999 also available in liposomes), and triethylenethiophosphoramide (thio-TEPA), with metho-trexate experience being by far the most substantial. Methotrexate is given at 6 mg/m^2 (maximum single dose of 15 mg) three times per week or until the CSF clears of malignant cells. Subsequently it is tapered off to once a week and then once a month for prophylaxis. An alternative schedule is 2 mg/m^2 for three days every two weeks, as developed by investigators at the National Cancer Institute (D. Poplack, personal communication).

Even though intrathecal administration of chemotherapeutic agents has become the standard of care for patients with a leptomeningeal malignancy, until recently (for liposomal cytarabine) there have been no control trials to demonstrate the superiority of this type of therapy over other routes of drug administration. There are obvious disadvantages to intrathecal therapy. The surgery for placement of an intrathecal reservoir and multiple lumbar punctures for drug instillation increase the risk of bleeding and infectious complications. Also, patients with CSF flow obstruction require an al-leviation of the block prior to the therapy. Other severe complications like myeloencephalopathy have occurred as a result of accidental overdose of intrathecal methotrexate [63]. A recent study by Glantz and coworkers [64] compared intrathecal methotrexate to high dose IV methotrexate. In that study 16 patients with solid tumor neoplastic meningitis received 1–4 courses of high dose ($8 \ g/m^2$) IV methotrexate with leucovorin rescue. Serum and CSF methotrexate levels were measured daily. Toxicity, response, and survival were compared to a reference group of 15 patients treated with standard intrathecal methotrexate during the same time interval. Median survival for the high dose IV methotrexate group was 13.8 months, with six patients still living 23.2 to 52.8 months after diagnosis. Of the eleven patients who have died, progressive leptomeningeal disease was the sole, or a major contributing, cause of death in six. Median survival for the intrathecal methotrexate group was 2.3 months. Of the 14 patients who have died, progressive leptomeningeal disease was the cause of death in eight. No significant toxicities, including hematological, were seen among the high dose IV methotrexate group. No patient discontinued therapy because of treatment-related side effects. CSF levels of methotrexate were 1×10^{-6} mol/l and were maintained for 48 hours. Concentrations above 1×10^{-8} mol/l persisted for more than six days. It is commonly acknowledged that concentration of 1×10^{-6} is effective for killing cancer cells, but concentrations as low as 1×10^{-8} mol/l can produce substantial tumor cell killing if exposure is long enough [65]. Authors also reported that CSF methotrexate concentrations were identical above and below CSF flow blocks in the two patients in whom that information was obtained. The minimal toxicity and the significant difference in survival time between the two non-randomized groups encouraged the authors to propose that until prospective studies are done, high dose IV methotrexate should be considered as a treatment of choice instead of intrathecal methotrexate for patients with non leukemic neoplastic meningitis provided there are no renal contraindications for administering high dose methotrexate.

Other indications

Methotrexate has had a prominent role in the treatment of breast cancer as part of combination regimens (e.g. CMF, CMFVP). Except for use in these combinations, MTX has been displaced from current use. Its analogue, edatrexate, is currently undergoing evaluation. Similarly, methotrexate has been used occasionally in soft tissue sarcomas. More recently, however, such use has nearly disappeared. Nevertheless, activity has recently been shown for edatrexate [66] and this may rekindle focus on this class of drugs. The effect of methotrexate on non small-cell lung cancer, colorectal cancer, and other gynecological cancers, such as cervix, has been minimal and it is unlikely that interest will reappear for this drug in these common adult solid tumors. The future for methotrexate and related drugs in the treatment of adult solid tumors is closely tied to a better understanding of factors predicting susceptibility to antifol-induced apoptosis, and to ways to enhance the selectivity of these drugs for tumor cells as opposed to normal tissues.

Principles of high dose methotrexate therapy

The rationale for using high dose methotrexate instead of a conventional dose is based on several considerations: 1) selective rescue of normal tissues vs. tumors, 2) the potential to overcome mechanisms of resistance such as impaired cellular uptake, dose-dependent increased formation of methotrexate polyglutamate derivatives (for fuller discussion refer to the chapter on methotrexate metabolism), and 3) the achievement of high concentrations of methotrexate in sanctuary sites, i.e. CSF, testicles, ovaries, and eyes. As has already been mentioned, high dose methotrexate therapy has an established role in some clinical situations. In children with ALL, administration of high dose methotrexate significantly lowered the systemic relapse rate in comparison to children who were treated with conventional doses of methotrexate [67]. High dose methotrexate as part of adjuvant multi-drug chemotherapy has been a part of regimens that helped decrease the two year relapse rate for osteosarcoma from 83% to 34% [68]. Recently, high dose IV methotrexate was also deemed superior to intrathecal methotrexate for leptomeningeal cancer [64], as mentioned above.

However, administration of high dose methotrexate poses significant risks requiring constant alertness on the part of the clinician. Several important principles have to be kept in mind in order to prevent toxicities such as severe myelosuppression, renal failure, mucositis, nausea, and diarrhea. For a detailed and excellent review of the subject refer to the article by Treon and Chabner [69].

Kidneys are the principal route of elimination for methotrexate. Glomerular filtration, tubular secretion, and tubular reabsorption all play a role in the renal handling of methotrexate. Patients considered for high dose methotrexate should have a normal serum creatinine concentration and a minimum glomerular filtration rate (GFR) of 60 ml/hour. In order to promote diuresis and to prevent the intra-tubular precipitation of methotrexate, the importance of aggressive hydration along with urine alkalinization cannot be overemphasized especially beyond moderate doses exceeding 300 mg/m^2. 7-OH-methotrexate is a metabolite not appreciably produced at a conventional dose of methotrexate [70, 71]. It has a limited aqueous solubility and may contribute to high dose methotrexate related renal toxicity. Methotrexate and 7-OH-methotrexate are 20 and 12 times more soluble at a pH of 7 than at a pH of 5, respectively [70]. One study showed that maintaining an alkaline urine pH is even more important than maintaining high urinary output for methotrexate clearance [71]. Urine alkalinity is usually maintained with IV or oral sodium bicarbonate. Monitoring serum methotrexate level is an essential part of high dose methotrexate administration. It is done in order to identify patients at the highest risk for methotrexate – related toxicity and delay in excretion is then coupled to enhanced leucovorin rescue. Administration of leucovorin usually starts 18–24 hours after the end of methotrexate infusion. Different schedules and doses of leucovorin have been adopted [71–75]. However, a key principle is to continue leucovorin rescue until serum methotrexate concentrations are <10 nmol/l, since higher concentrations inhibit bone marrow proliferation [65, 76].

Also, it is important to avoid drugs that can potentially displace methotrexate from serum proteins. Such drugs include salicylates, phenylbutazone, phenytoin, and sulfonamides. Non-steroidal anti-inflammatory drugs should especially be avoided since, in addition to displacing methotrexate from serum proteins, they can inhibit its renal clearance. Other drugs that should be avoided include probenecid, which inhibits renal tubular transport of methotrexate. Concomitant or preceding use of nephrotoxic drugs such as gentamicin and cisplatin represent a potential threat, since they may radically change the tolerance of a dose of methotrexate that was previously safe. In patients with ascites or pleural effusions it is advisable to drain those effusions first. It has been shown [77, 78] that the plasma half-life of methotrexate was prolonged in patients with third-spacing of fluids. This is a result of sustained back diffusion of methotrexate to the vasculature from the third-space fluids where high concentrations of methotrexate can accumulate.

In summary, careful patient selection, adequate hydration, urinary alkalinization, avoidance of drug interactions, and drainage of third-space fluids can prevent most of the toxicities that can be potentially associated with administration of high dose methotrexate. However, repeated courses within intricate chemotherapeutic regimens continue to be associated with occasional life-threatening toxicities that require careful risk/benefit consideration before widespread adoption.

References

1 Kennedy A (1995) Persistent nonmetastatic gestational trophoblastic disease. *Semin Oncol* 22 (2): 161–165
2 Isonishi S, Terashima Y (1996) Methotrexate in gynecologic oncology. *Jap J Cancer chemo* 23 (14): 1896–1900
3 Homesley H (1998) Single-agent therapy for nonmetastatic and low-risk gestational trophoblastic disease. *J Repro Med* 43 (1): 69–74
4 Roberts J, Lurain J (1996) Treatment of low risk gestational trophoblastic tumors with single-agent chemotherapy. *Amer J Obstet Gynecol* 174 (6): 1917–1924
5 Newlands E, Bower M, Holden L, Short D, Seckl MJ, Rustin GJ, Begent RH, Bagshawe KD (1998) Management of resistant gestational trophoblastic tumors. *Journal of Reproductive Medicine* 43 (2): 111–118
6 Lurain J (1998) Management of high-risk gestational trophoblastic disease. *J Repro Med* 43 (1): 44–52
7 Santillana S, Mariategui J, Mas L, Velarde C, Casanova L, Carracedo C, Valdivia S, Gomez H, Otero J, Rodrigues W, Vallejos C (1995) Comparison of two classification systems for metastatic gestational trophoblastic disease: substratification for high-risk patients. *Proc Am Soc Clin Oncol* 14: A768
8 Hartenbach E, Saltzman A, Carter J, Twiggs L (1995) A novel strategy using G-CSF to support EMA/CO for high-risk gestational trophoblastic disease. *Gynecol Oncol* 56 (1): 105–108, 1995.

9 Bower M, Newlands E, Holden L, Short D, Brock C, Rustin GJ, Begent RH, Bagshawe KD (1997) EMA/CO for high-risk gestational trophoblastic tumors: results from a cohort of 272 patients. *J Clin Oncol* 15 (7): 2636–2643

10 Soto-Wright V, Goldstein DP, Bernstein MR, Berkowitz RS (1997) The management of gestational trophoblastic tumors with etoposide, methotrexate, and actinomycin D. *Gynecol Oncol* 64 (1): 156–159

11 Rustin G, Newlands E, Lutz J, Holden L, Bagshawe KD, Hiscox JG, Foskett M, Fuller S, Short D (1996) Combination but not single-agent chemotherapy for gestational tropho-blastic tumors increases the incidence of second tumors. *J Clin Oncol* 14 (10): 2769–2773

12 Newlands E, Rustin G, Lutz JM, Holden L, Bagshawe KD, Hiscox JG, Bell J (1995) Chemotherapy for gestational trophoblastic tumors may increase the incidence of second tumors and may cause premature menopause. *Proc Am Soc Clin Oncol* 14: A744

13 Brinkley W, Torti F (1997) Systemic Chemotherapy of transitional cell carcinoma of the urothelium. *Semin Surg Oncol* 13 (5): 365–375

14 Roth BJ (1995) Palliative chemotherapy in advanced bladder cancer. *Semin Oncol* 22 (2): 10–15

15 Roth BJ, Bajorin DF (1995) Advanced bladder cancer: the need to identify new agents in the post M-VAC world. *J Urol* 153: 894–900

16 Loehrer PJ Sr, Einhorn LH, Elson PJ, Crawford ED, Kuebler J, Tannock I, Rag-havan D, Stuart-Harris R, Sarosdy MF, Lowe BA, et al (1992) A randomized com-parison of cisplatin alone or in combination with methotrexate, vinblastine, and doxo-rubicin in patients with metastatic urothelial carcinoma: A cooperative group study [published erratum appears in *J Clin Oncol* 11 (2): 384, 1993]. *J Clin Oncol* 10 (7): 1066–1073

17 Saxman SB, Propert KJ, Einhorn LH, Crawford ED, Tannock I, Raghavan D, Loehrer PJ Sr, Trump D (1997) Long-term follow-up of a phase III intergroup study of cisplatin alone or in combination with methotrexate, vinblastine, and doxorubicin in patients with metastatic urothelial carcinoma: a cooperative group study. *J Clin Oncol* 15 (7): 2564–2569

18 Harker W, Meyers F, Freiha F, Palmer JM, Shortliffe LD, Hannigan JF, McWhirter KM, Torti FM (1985) Cisplatin, methotrexate, and vinblastine (CMV): an effective chemotherapy regimen for metastatic transitional cell carcinoma of the urinary tract. A Northern California Oncology Group study. *J Clin Oncol* 3: 1463–1470

19 Rosenberg S, Williams R (1987) Cis-platinum, methotrexate, and vinblastine (CMV) for advanced carcinoma of the bladder and upper urinary tract. *J Urol* 137: A157

20 Fagbemi S, Stadler W (1998) New chemotherapy regimens for advanced bladder cancer. *Semin Urol Oncol* 16 (1): 23–29

21 Logothetis CJ, Dexeus FH, Finn L, Sella A, Amato RJ, Ayala AG, Kilbourn RG (1990) A prospective randomized trial comparing MVAC and CISCA chemotherapy for patients with metastatic urothelial tumors. *J Clin Oncol* 8: 1050–1055

22 Herr HW, Scher HI (1994) Neoadjuvant chemotherapy and partial cystectomy for invasive bladder cancer. *J Clin Oncol* 12: 975–980

23 Hall RR (1996) Neoadjuvant CMV chemotherapy and cystectomy or radiotherapy in muscle invasive bladder cancer. First analysis of MRC/EORTC intercontinental trial. *Proc Am Soc Clin Oncol* 15: A612

24 Tu SM, Hossan E, Amato R, Kilbourn R, Logothetis CJ (1995) Paclitaxel, cisplatin, and methotrexate combination chemotherapy is active in the treatment of refractory urothelial malignancies. *J Urol* 154: 1719–1722

25 Klein H (1989) Long term results with FAMTX (5- fluorouracil, Adriamycin, methotrexate) in advanced gastric cancer. *Cancer Res* 9: 1025

26 Murad AM, Santiago FF, Petroianu A, Rocha PR, Rodrigues MA, Rausch M (1993) Modified therapy with 5-fluorouracil, doxorubicin, and methotrexate in advanced gastric cancer. *Cancer* 72: 37–41

27 Kelsen D, Atiq O, Saltz L, Toomasi F, Trochanowski B, Niedzwiecki D (1991) FAMTX (fluorouracil, methotrexate, adriamycin) is as effective and less toxic than EAP (etoposide, adriamycin, cisplatin): a random assigned trial in gastric cancer. *Proc Am Soc Clin Oncol* 10: 137

28 Wils JA, Klein HO, Wagener DJT, Bleiberg H, Reis H, Korsten F, Conroy T, Fickers M, Leyvraz S, Buyse M et al (1991) Sequential high dose methotrexate and fluorouracil combined with doxorubicin – a step ahead in the treatment of advanced gastric cancer: a trial

of the European Organization for Reasearch and Treatment of Cancer Gastointestinal Tract Cooperative Group. *J Clin Oncol* 9: 827–831

29 Webb A, Cunningham D, Scarffe JH, Harper P, Norman A, Joffe JK, Hughes M, Mansi J, Findlay M, Hill A et al. (1997) Randomized trial comparing epirubicin, cisplatin, and fluorouracil vs. fluorouracil, doxorubicin, and methotrexate in advanced esophagogastric cancer. *J Clin Oncol* 15 (1): 261–267

30 Woods RL, Fox RM, Tattersall MHN (1981) Methotrexate treatment of head and neck cancers: a dose response evaluation. *Cancer Treat Rep* 65: 155–159

31 Taylor SG, McGuire WP, Hauck WW, Showel JL, Lad TE (1984) A randomized comparison of high-dose infusion methotrexate vs. standard dose weekly therapy in head and neck squamous cancer. *J Clin Oncol* 2: 1006–1011

32 DeConti RC, Schoenfeld D (1981) A randomized prospective comparison of intermittent methotrexate, methotrexate with leucovorin, and a methotrexate combination in head and neck cancers. *Cancer* 48: 1061–1072

33 Forastiere AA, Metch B, Schuller DE, Ensley JF, Hutchins LF, Triozzi P, Kish JA, McClure S, VonFeldt E, Williamson SK, et al (1992) Randomized comparison of cisplatin plus fluorouracil and carboplatin plus fluorouracil vs. methotrexate in advanced squamous-cell carcinoma of the head and neck: A Southwest Oncology Group Study. *J Clin Oncol* 10 (8): 1245–1251

34 De Angelis LM, Yahalom J, Thaler HT, Kher U (1992) Combined modality treatment for primary CNS lymphoma. *J Clin Oncol* 10: 635–643

35 Gabbai AA, Hochberg FH, Lingood RM, Bashir R, Hotleman K (1989) High dose methotrexate for non-AIDS primary central nervous system lymphoma. *J Neurosurg* 190: 70

36 Loeffler JS, Ervin TJ Mauch P, Skarin A, Weinstein HJ, Canellos G, Cassady JR (1985) Primary lymphomas of the central nervous system: patterns of failures and factors that influence survival. *J Clin Oncol* 3: 490–494

37 Glass J, Gruber ML, Cher L, Hochberg FH (1994) Preirradiation methotrexate chemotherapy of primary central nervous system lymphoma: long term outcome. *J Neurosurg* 81:188–195

38 Freilich RJ, Delattre JY, De Angelis LM (1996) Chemotherapy without radiation therapy as initial treatment for primary central nervous system lymphoma in older patients. *Neurology* 46: 435–439

39 Dahlberg SA, Henner WD, Crossen JR, Tableman M, Petrillo A, Braziel R, Neuwelt EA (1996) Non-AIDS primary CNS lymphoma: First example of durable response in a primary brain tumor using enhanced chemotherapy without cognitive loss and without radiotherapy. *Cancer J Sci Am* 2: 166–174

40 O'Brien PC, Roos DE, Liew KH, Trotter GE, Barton MB, Walker QJ, Poulsen MG, Olver IN (1996) Preliminary results of combined chemotherapy and radiotherapy for non-AIDS primary central nervous system lymphoma. Trans-Tasman Radiation Oncology Group (TROG). *Med J Aust* 166 (8): 424–427

41 Abrey LE, De Angelis LM, Yahalom J (1998) Long term survival in primary CNS lymphoma. *J Clin Oncol* 16 (3): 859–863

42 De Angelis LM, De lattre JY, Posner JB (1989) Radiation induced dementia in patients cured of brain metastasis. *Neurology* 39: 789–796

43 Duffey P, Chari G, Cartlidge NE, Shaw PJ (1996) Progressive deterioration of intelect and motor function occurring several decades after cranial irradiation. *Arch Neurol* 53: 814–818

44 Crossen JR, Garwood D, Glatstein E, Neuwelt EA (1994) Neurobehavioral sequelae of cranial irradiation in adults: A review of radiation induced encephalopathy. *J Clin Oncol* 12: 627–42

45 De Angelis LM, Yahalom J (1997) Primary Central Nervous System Lymphoma. In: De Vita VT, Hellman S, Rosenberg SA (eds): *Cancer: Principles and Practice of Oncology,* 5th edition 2233–2242

46 Magrath I, Adde M, Shad A (1996) Adults and children with small non-cleaved-cell lymphoma have a similar excellent outcome when treated with the same chemotherapy regimen. J *Clin Oncol* 14 (3): 925–934

47 Soussain C, Patte C, Ostronoff M, Delmer A, Rigal-Huguet F, Cambier N, Leprise PY, Francois S, Cony-Makhoul P, Harousseau JL et al (1995) Small noncleaved cell lymphoma in adults. A retrospective study of 65 adults treated with LMB pediatrics protocols. *Blood* 85 (3): 664–674

48 Jaffe M, Patel S, Benjamin R (1995) Chemotherapy in osteosarcoma. *Hematol Oncol Clin North Am* 9 (4): 825–840

49 Bruland OS, Pihl A (1997) On the current management of osteosarcoma, a critical evaluation and proposal for a modified treatment strategy. *Eur J Cancer* 33 (11): 7125–1731

50 Picci P, Bacci G, Baldini N, Mercuri M, Briccoli A (1995) Introduction to sarcomas. 2nd EORTC International Hong Kong Symposium on Currents Trends in Cancer Care, February 13–15, Hong Kong, 33 abstract

51 Ferrari S, Bacci G, Picci P, Mercuri M, Briccoli A, Pinto D, Gasbarrini A, Tienghi A (1997) Long-term follow-up and post-relapse survival in patients with non-metastatic osteosarcoma of the extremity treated with neoadjuvant chemotherapy. *Ann Oncol* 8 (8): 765–771

52 Kawai A, Sugihara S, Kunisada T, Hamada M, Inoue H (1996) The importance of doxorubicin and methotrexate dose intensity in the chemotherapy of osteosarcoma. Archives of Orthopaedic & Trauma Surgery 115 (2): 68–70

53 Delepine N, Delepine G, Bacci G, Rosen G, Desbois JC (1996) Influence of methotrexate dose intensity on outcome of patients with high grade osteogenic osteosarcoma. Analysis of the literature. *Cancer* 78 (10): 2127–2135

54 Delepine N, Cornille H, Delepine G, Desbois JC (1995) Meta analysis of methotrexate outcome for patients with osteogenic osteosarcoma. *Anticancer Res* 15 (5A): 1715–1716

55 Delepine N, Delepine G, Cornille H, Brion F, Arnaud P, Desbois JC (1995) Dose escalation with pharmacokinetics monitoring in methotrexate chemotherapy of osteosarcoma. *Anticancer Res* 15 (2): 489–494

56 Bacci G, Ferrari S, Delepine N, Bertoni F, Picci P, Mercuri M, Bacchini P, Brach del Prever A, Tienghi A, Comandone A, Campanacci M (1998) Predictive factors of histologic response to primary chemotherapy in osteosarcoma of the extremity: study of 272 patients preoperatively treated with high dose methotrexate, doxorubicin, and cisplatin. *J Clin Oncol* 16 (2): 658–663

57 Bacci G, Ferrari S, Picci P, Zolezzi C, Gherlinzoni F, Iantorno D, Cazzola A (1996) Methotrexate serum concentration and histological response to multiagent primary chemotherapy for osteosarcoma of the limbs. *J Chemother* 8 (6): 472–478

58 Meyers PA, Gorlick R, Heller G, Casper E, Lane J, Huvos AG, Healey JH (1998) Intensification of preoperative chemotherapy for osteogenic sarcoma: results of the Memorial Sloan-Kettering (T12) protocol. *J Clin Oncol* 16 (7): 2452–2458

59 Bacci G, Mercuri M, Briccolo A, Ferrari S, Bertoni F, Donati D, Monti C, Zanoni A, Forni C, Manfrini M (1997) Osteogenic sarcoma of the extremity with detectable lung metastases at presentation. Results of treatment of 23 patients with chemotherapy followed by simultaneous resection of primary and metastatic lesions. *Cancer* 79 (2): 245–254

60 Miser J, Arndt C, Smithson W, Gilchrist G, Edmonson J, Sim F, Rock M, Pritchard D, Shives T, Wold L (1998) Long term follow-up of high grade osteosarcoma treated with preoperative ifosfamide, adriamycin, and high dose methotrexate with cisplatinum added postop for poor responders. *Proc Am Soc Clin Onc* 17: 2054

61 Hosain F, Spencer RP, Couthon, Sturtz GL (1996) Targeted delivery of antineoplastic agent to bone: biodistribution studies of tecnetium-99m-labeled gem-bisphosphonate conjugate of methotrexate. *J Nucl Med* 37 (1): 105–107

62 Li WW, Fan J, Bertino JR (1996) Overexpression of p21 mediates increased sensitivity to methotrexate, tomudex, and doxorubicin in a human osteosarcoma cell line. *Proc Am Assoc Cancer Res* 37: A2177

63 Spiegel RJ, Cooper PR, Blum RH, Speyer JL, McBride D, Mangiardi J (1984) Treatment of massive intrathecal methotrexate overdose by ventriculolumbar perfusion. *N Engl J Med* 311 (16): 386–388

64 Glantz M, Cole BF, Recht L, Akerley W, Mills P, Saris S, Hochberg F, Calabresi P, Egorin MJ (1998) High dose intravenous methotrexate for patients with non leukemic leptomeningeal cancer: Is intrathecal chemotherapy necessary? *J Clin Oncol* 16 (4): 1561–1567

65 Chabner BA, Young R (1973) Threshold methotrexate concentration for *in vivo* inhibition of DNA synthesis in normal and tumorous target tissues. *J Clin Invest* 52: 1804–1811

66 Freeman AI, Weinberg V, Brecher M, Jones B, Glicksman AS, Sinks LF, Weil M, Pleuss H, Hananian J, Burgert EO Jr et al (1983) Comparison of intermediate dose methotrexate with cranial irradiation for the post induction treatment of acute lymphocytic leukemia in children. *N Engl J Med* 308: 477–484

67 Wasserheit C, Blum R, Ryan L (1998) Phase II trial of Edatrexate in adult patients with metastatic soft tissue sarcomas, an ECOG Phase II Trial. *Proc Am Soc Clin Onc* 17: 1978a

68 Jaffe N, Link MP, Cohen D, Traggis D, Frei E 3d, Watts H, Beardsley GP, Abelson HT (1981) High dose methotrexate in osteogenic sarcoma. *Natl Cancer Inst Monogr* 56: 201–206

69 Treon SP, Chabner BA (1996) Concepts in use of high-dose methotrexate therapy: *Clin Chem* 42 (8): 1322–1329

70 Jacobs SA, Stoller RG, Chabner BA, Johns DJ (1976) 7-hydroxymethotrexate as a urinary metabolite in human subjects and rhesus monkeys receiving high dose methotrexate. *J Clinic Invest* 57: 534–538

71 Jacobs SA, Stoller RG, Chabner BA, Johns DG (1977) Dose dependent metabolism of methotrexate in man and rhesus monkeys. *Cancer Treat Rep* 61: 651–656

72 Skarin AT, Zuckerman KS, Pitman SW, Rosenthal DS, Moloney W, Frei E 3d, Canellos GP (1977) High-dose methotrexate with folinic acid in the treatment of advanced non-Hodgkin lymphoma including CNS involvement. *Blood* 50: 1039–1047

73 Jaffe N, Robertson R, Ayala A, et al (1985) Comparison intraarterial cis-diamminedichloro-platinum with high dose methotrexate and citrovorum factor rescue in the treatment of primary osteosarcoma. *J Clin Oncol* 3: 1101–1104

74 Isacoff WH, Morrison PF, Aroesty J (1977) Pharmacokinetics of high-dose methotrexate with citrovorum factor rescue. *Cancer Treat Rep* 61: 1665–1674

75 Goldin A, Venditti JM, Kline I (1966) Eradication of leukaemic cells (L1210) by metho-trexate and methotrexate plus citrovorum factor. *Nature* 212: 1548–1550

76 Adamson PC, Balis FM, Mccully CL, Godwin KS, Bacher JD, Walsh TJ, Poplack DG (1991) Rescue of experimental intrathecal methotrexate overdose with carboxypeptidase-G2. *J Clin Oncol* 9: 670–674

77 Fox RM (1979) Methotrexate nephrotoxicity. *Clin Exp Pharmacol Physiol* 5: 43–44

78 Wan SH, Huffman DH, Azarnoff DL, Stephens R, Hoogstraten B (1974) Effect of route of administration and effusions on methotrexate pharmacokinetics. *Cancer Res* 34: 3487–3491

Methotrexate
ed. by B. N. Cronstein und J. R. Bertino
© 2000 Birkhäuser Verlag Basel/Switzerland

The use of methotrexate in the treatment of childhood malignancies

Barton A. Kamen and Richard I. Drachtman

Cancer Institute of New Jersey, 195 Little Albany Street, New Brunswick, NJ 08901, USA

Introduction

The modern era of chemotherapy for patients with cancer began fifty years ago when Farber et al. reported on the use of aminopterin to induce a temporary remission in acute lymphoblastic leukemia in children [1]. Although aminopterin is not in common usage at this time, folic acid antagonists remain amongst the most widely used antineoplastic agents. Methotrexate is the most frequently used drug of this group and is a mainstay in the treatment of common childhood malignancies. It is an integral component of therapy for patients being treated for acute lympho-blastic leukemia and Non-Hodgkin's Lymphoma and is often used in the treatment of patients with osteogenic sarcoma.

Given the immense literature concerning methotrexate (>25,000 citations in medlines) and the content of other chapters in this book, it is not the intent of this chapter to present a comprehensive treatise, but rather to review current issues, which may be unique to children, such as drug dosing, scheduling, metabolism, and problems of resistance and toxicity. Furthermore, although there are numerous reports of the activity of methotrexate in the treatment of a number of different diseases, only those for which it is a standard part of therapy will be emphasized. We have chosen to cite some of the classic and more current literature since there are recent texts and articles already providing comprehensive reviews [2, 3] Omissions of citations to pertinent work is due to space. The authors, as pediatric oncologists gratefully acknowledge colleagues who are clinical investigators and/or workers in the anti-folate field.

Pharmacology

Before proceeding with a summary of the use of methotrexate in pediatric patients with cancer and at the risk of being somewhat redundant with other chapters in this text, a brief reminder about the pharmacology of the drug will be provided here. The goal is to place in perspective the pharmacology of methotrexate with the physiology/biochemistry of folic acid. Methotrexate is a folate analog. It shares many of the same pathways for transport, metabolism and catabolism. As an organic acid it also has some unique pathways for secretion (e.g. multi-organic acid transporters in both the proximal renal tubule and bile canalicular membranes (MOATs)). Thus the basic pharmacodynamics of methotrexate should be related to the overall homeostasis of folates. This relationship provides a firm foundation for understanding and improving the therapeutic efficacy of the drug (reviewed in [4]).

Folic acid is a water soluble vitamin which is a co-factor or substrate in a number of important metabolic reactions. The fully reduced species, tetrahydrofolate, carries a one carbon group for the *de novo* synthesis of purines and thymidine, the conversion of homocysteine to methionine and the general maintenance of adequate methyl groups for 1-carbon metabolism (i.e. synthesis of S-adenosylmethionine). The clinical features of a folate deficiency have been recognized for more than 50 years. These include megaloblastic anemia, epithelial dysplasias, birth defects (especially neural tube abnormalities) and most recently a critical relationship between folate and increased risk of vascular disease. Biochemically, these defects are likely due to mis-incorporation of deoxyuridine (instead of thymidine) into DNA, abnormal methylation of DNA bases, decreased purine synthesis or an increased concentration of homocysteine, the latter which may be the cause of vascular disease (reviewed in [5, 6]).

The recognition that folate is both an important anti-anemia factor and that folate supplementation will accelerate the growth of leukemia cells over 50 years ago, years before the target enzymes for methotrexate and even the synthetic pathways for purine and pyrimidine synthesis had been completely elucidated, was the rationale for the development of folate analogs as cytotoxic drugs [7]. The subsequent decades have witnessed the development of many folate analogs with specific intracellular targets other than dihydrofolic acid reductase (e.g. thymidylate synthase, and the *de novo* synthesis of purines, i.e. glycinamide ribonucleotide (GAR) and aminoimidazole-4-carboxamide ribonucleotide (AICAR) transformylase), but as of yet none have replaced methotrexate. Recently we have initiated clinical trials of aminopterin based upon laboratory data showing it to be a better substrate than methotrexate for folylpolyglutamate synthetase (FPGS) and 50 years of hindsight into empirical scheduling, dosing and overall efficacy of methotrexate [8, 9].

Since folate is a vitamin (a vital amine that cannot be synthesized under usual conditions) the body's conservation of folate is extremely high. Even during the stress of pregnancy, the recommended daily allowance (RDA) is only 400 µg/day. Folate accumulation by most cells is via a non-concentrative, bidirectional system, the reduced folate carrier (RFC) which is topologically similar to organic acid transporters. Recent studies of lymphoblasts obtained at the time of diagnosis reveal an approximately 100 – fold range in RNA expression assessed by PCR [10]. The vitamin is trapped in the cell by addition of gamma-glutamyl side chains by the enzyme folylpolyglutamate synthetase (FPGS) which appears to be a cycle (growth) – dependent enzyme [11, 12]. In order to prevent renal loss of folate and to package and concentrate folate in specific compartments (e.g. fetus and cerebrospinal fluid) there are also specific receptors on the brush border of the proximal tubules, on the choroid plexus and syncytiotropho-blast cells which ensure the conservation of folate [13, reviewed in 14]. Alterations in the quantity or function of any of these proteins by mutation or natural polymorphisms could result in resistance to, or an increased toxicity of, methotrexate [6, 15–17].

Acute lymphoblastic leukemia

Acute lymphoblastic leukemia is the most common malignancy in child-hood e.g. approximately 2200 cases diagnosed each year in the United States [18]. As a result of multi-institutional clinical trials and laboratory research under the auspices of co-operative groups all over the world, the mortality of childhood acute lymphoblastic leukemia has declined drama-tically since the first report of the use of aminopterin [1]. In a recent editorial, Dr. Joseph Simone noted that the remarkable success in treatment of children with acute lymphoblastic leukemia during the last 20–25 years has come without the addition of any major new drugs [19]. Specifically, the mortality rate for children with acute lymphoblastic leukemia has decreased from 1.3 to 0.4/100,000 in the last 25 years and methotrexate, 6-mercaptopurine, vincristine, steroids and asparaginase were developed in the 1950s and 1960s. In the present era the majority of patients with child-hood acute lymphoblastic leukemia are curable, with the survival rate of patients with 'standard risk' leukemia approaching ninety percent by some estimates. Methotrexate, although less potent than its predecessor aminop-terin, had greater efficacy in animal studies [20–22] and has been an integral part of childhood acute lymphoblastic leukemia regimens since 1961 when Frei and colleagues published the results of a multi-institutio-nal study of methotrexate and 6-mercaptopurine which showed definitively the benefits of anti-metabolite therapy [23].

Although methotrexate remains an integral part of therapy for acute lymphoblastic leukemia, the optimal method of administration, scheduling and dosing are still controversial (earlier literature reviewed in [24]). The choice of scheduling and dosing will not only impact cure rate but also the toxicity profile, which will be detailed later. Methotrexate is typically used in the continuation phase (also referred to as a maintenance phase in earlier literature) of most current protocols. Specifically, treatment of children with acute lymphoblastic leukemia is initiated with an induction phase consisting of a vinca alkaloid, a corticosteroid, asparaginase and often an anthracycline. More than 95% of children will achieve a remission within four weeks. Following induction of a remission, there is a period referred to as a re-induction or intensification phase, in which chemotherapy more intensive than that used in continuation therapy is applied to 'make the remission better,' i.e. kill cells we cannot detect. This time period is often when an intensive central nervous system prophylaxis is also initiated (see below). Following this, continuation therapy of 2–3 years duration and primarily anti-metabolite based is instituted. Methotrexate is a cornerstone of maintenance therapy and is administered orally, intramuscularly, intravenously or intrathecally.

As is well known, methotrexate is unique among chemotherapy agents, in that there is a specific antidote, folate (usually leucovorin (leukovorin), 5-formyltetrahydrofolic acid). This has allowed a remarkable increase in the dose of methotrexate to be used (reviewed in [24, 25]). Doses in excess of 30 g/m^2 have been administered to children. Since as noted earlier, the daily requirement of the vitamin is only 400 µg, this represents a dose of drug that is more than 70,000 times the RDA for the vitamin. Despite the intuitive notion that the physiology of folate (i.e. homeostasis) should be related to the pharmacology of an analog which shares uptake, metabolism and catabolism pathways and that should suggest a limit to a dose, these larger doses have been utilized and seem to improve outcome in some, but not all studies [26–28]. The pharmacokinetic analysis of these studies revealed a marked (4–6 fold) inter-patient variability in drug clearance (reviewed in [3]). Multiple courses of intermediate dose (approximately 500 mg/m^2) in a phase III trial for treatment of children with acute lymphoblastic leukemia was pioneered more than 15 years ago [29]. The goal was to decrease relapse, especially in the CNS, by increasing methotrexate concentration in the CSF. Larger doses > 1000 mg/m^2 as a short 2–4 h infusion or 24 h infusion are still incorporated into phase III trials. In comparing these regimens it is important to note that the number of courses of methotrexate and the timing and dosing of the leukovorin are not standardized. Abromowitch et al. [30] suggested that there may be a correlation between higher serum levels of methotrexate and improved outcome. A more recent Pediatric Oncology Group (POG) study compared intensification with intermediate-dose intravenous methotrexate with intravenous mercaptopurine to repetitive low dose oral methotrexate with intravenous mercaptopurine for children with lower risk B lineage acute lymphoblastic leukemia [31]. This study found that intensification with 1000 mg methotrexate/m^2 as a 24 h infusion was marginally superior to 30 mg methotrexate/m^2 every six hours (six doses, total dose of 180 mg/m^2). However, on closer examination, since the same dose of leukovorin rescue was used despite the fact that the dose of methotrexate differed ten-fold (methotrexate is only 30–50% bio-available) this study may have shown that too much methotrexate and too much leukovorin are given [32]. Of note is that toxicity in the higher dose (IV) group was significant [31, 33]. Moreover, although it did not reach statistical significance there were approximately twice as many CNS relapses in the group treated with oral methotrexate (approximately 93% vs. 96% protection). This may be due to selective accumulation of folate in the CNS via a receptor-mediated process on the choroid plexus which has a much larger affinity for folate than methotrexate. Specifically, only 5 mg of oral leukovorin several hours before a scheduled spinal tap was found to nearly triple CSF folate [34]. What would 10–15 mg leukovorin/m^2/dose times five doses do to CSF folate? In comparison, our institution has been using divided dose, oral methotrexate (25 mg/m^2/dose times four doses on a weekly or every other week schedule) with only 5 mg leukovorin/m^2/dose given 12 and 24 h after the last dose of methotrexate as the major component of continuation therapy. 322 patients have been treated and 180 are > 5 years off therapy. The event-free survivals of the standard risk and high risk patients are 90% ± 2% and 81% ± 2% respectively (Winick and Kamen, unpublished observations). In light of the CNS disease noted above, we have seen more isolated CNS relapses than marrow failures. Maybe there is a small group that could benefit from more intense central nervous system prophylaxis?

Augmented post-induction therapy has been shown to improve the outcome of 'higher risk' children who also had a poor early response to induction therapy [35]. The augmented regimen in this study included more vincristine, asparaginase, methotrexate and dexamethasone than the standard regimen, while the standard regimen included more oral prednisone, methotrexate and mercaptopurine. It is unclear which individual agents were most important for patients in the augmented arm, but the most significant increases were in the intensity of the methotrexate and asparaginase arm during the "Capizzi regimen" of therapy as shown in Table 1 [36].

Table 1. Comparison of the dose intensity of a standard and augmented arm of therapy of a children's cancer group study for children with high-risk acute lymphoblastic leukemia*

Drug	Standard	Augmented	A/S
	(mg or units/m^2/first 53 weeks)		
Prednisone	1815	900	0.5
Cyclophosphamide	3000	4000	1.33
Mercaptopurine	21600	7980	0.37
Vincristine	27	40.5	1.5
Cytarabine	1800	2400	1.33
Asparaginase	36000	366000	10.0
Methotrexate	660	2210	6–10**
Dexamethasone	270	540	2.0
Doxorubicin	75	150	2.0
Thioguanine	840	1680	2.0

* The data is compiled from the information presented in detail in reference [35].
** Since the methotrexate in the standard arm is given PO but IV in the intensive phases of the augmented arm, the absolute ratio is more likely in the 6–10 range because of issues of bioavailability.

Balis et al. recently assessed the pharmacokinetics of methotrexate in a homogenous population of lower risk patients with acute lymphoblastic leukemia and correlated pharmacokinetic parameters with disease outcome [37]. Plasma drug concentrations were highly variable with significant intra-patient variability and did not distinguish patients with higher rates of relapse. However, data has been presented by Evans et al. who individualized therapy in the remission phase of acute lymphoblastic leukemia therapy (containing high-dose methotrexate, teniposide and cytarabine) on the basis of drug clearance as opposed to using plasma concentrations and concluded that normalization can improve outcome [38]. It seems intuitively correct that normalizing kinetics (e.g. eliminating a large variation in methotrexate pharmacokinetics) will improve overall results for a specific protocol. The larger issue is whether the number of doses, the scheduling and the actual dose and how much leukovorin are given are optimal. For example, it has been shown that there is a decrease in metabolism of methotrexate to a polyglutamate species by freshly isolated lymphoblasts incubated with [^{3}H]-methotrexate as the concentration of drug was increased from 1 to 50 µM *in vitro* [39].

Goals for the future use of methotrexate in childhood acute lymphoblastic leukemia are multi-faceted and must take into account short term and, more importantly, long term toxicity (see below). First, it is critical to determine the optimal dosing and method of administration of methotrexate to assure the greatest efficacy. This requires addressing issues of patient compliance and adequate identification of patients who may benefit from alternative methods of administration, such as the intramuscular route [40]. The role of individualized dosing remains controversial at this time. Current ongoing studies by the co-operative groups in Europe and the United States are addressing this issue. Second, it is also important to consider the role of other agents and their interaction with methotrexate; it is difficult to specifically determine the role of methotrexate alone when given as part of an intensive poly-pharmaceutical approach to leukemia and is synergistic with thiopurines such as 6-mercaptopurine and 6-thioguanine. Third, baseline folate and use of leukovorin are likely to be significant prognostic factors based upon information provided earlier and the current lack of standardized 'high-dose' methotrexate and leukovorin rescue, the former having a 6-8 fold variation in pharmacokinetic parameters and the latter not being standardized as to timing and total dose.

Central nervous system therapy

The central nervous system (CNS) has been noted as a 'sanctuary site' for leukemia since effective treatment for obtaining and maintaining remission has been available. One of the earliest reports of CNS leukemic relapse occurred in two patients treated with methotrexate, cortisone and adrenocortitropic hormone (ACTH) in 1954 [41]. These children developed obesity and neurological symptoms and were noted to have lymphoblasts in the cerebrospinal fluid. They were subsequently treated with intrathecal methotrexate, albeit with only a partial response. Animal studies and further clinical work with children shortly thereafter firmly established the use of intrathecal methotrexate for the treatment of CNS involvement with acute lymphoblastic leukemia (reviewed in [24]). The next logical step was the establishment of multimodality or total therapy which included the use of specific CNS prophylaxis in the form of radiation therapy with or without intrathecal methotrexate [42].

The incidence of CNS relapse ranges from 5% to 8% in most studies over the past decade. Concern with regard to the side effects of cranial irradiation, in particular the occurrence of secondary brain tumors and cognitive defects, has led to various strategies to decrease the use of radiation. One of these strategies has been the intensification of intrathecal therapy. Pui et al. have reported on the use of early intensification of intrathecal chemotherapy with methotrexate, cytarabine and hydrocortisone in a successful attempt to reserve cranial irradiation only for higher risk patients [43]. This manuscript also provides an excellent literature list.

Other developments in acute lymphoblastic leukemia treatment may enable clinicians to further tailor the individual need for cranial irradiation while continuing treatment with systemic and intrathecal therapy. These include the observation that dexamethasone may penetrate the CSF better than prednisolone [44]. Current ongoing Phase III studies in the Children's Cancer Group are notable for the elimination of cranial irradiation for all patients except those with overt CNS disease or those who are slow responders, that is those that are not in bone marrow remission by day seven of induction. The role of triple intrathecal therapy (TIT, cytarabine, methotrexate and hydrocortisone) vs. single-agent intrathecal therapy with methotrexate also needs to be more fully evaluated from an efficacy point of view.

With the increasing use of intrathecal methotrexate, as well as the use of higher doses of methotrexate that may penetrate the blood brain barrier in an attempt to avoid cranial irradiation, and provide better control of systemic disease, the neurotoxicity of methotrexate has become increasingly evident. Of particular concern is the development of chronic demyelinating encephalopathy in children with consequent cognitive issues [45]. Issues of neurotoxicity are addressed more completely below.

Non-Hodgkin's lymphoma

As the efficacy of methotrexate in the treatment of leukemia has evolved, the activity of methotrexate was also established for the treatment of lymphoma. Many chemotherapy regimens for lymphoblastic lymphoma have been based on protocols initially intended for the treatment of acute lymphoblastic leukemia. Most widely used protocols are variants of the LSA2L2 regimen of which intermediate-dose methotrexate in the range of 1000 mg/m² is an integral feature. Variations of the cyclophosphamide, oncovin, methotrexate, prednisone (COMP) regimen with methotrexate in the range of 300 mg/m² are commonly used in cases of lymphoblastic lymphoma with more limited disease. Intrathecal methotrexate is also used for CNS prophylaxis in both of these regimens [46, 47]. Treatment of small non-cleaved cell lymphoma in childhood is typically based on alkylating agents, but methotrexate is often a part of these regimens as well. Concerns regarding the toxicity of methotrexate and a need for optimal dosing in the treatment of Non-Hodgkin's Lymphoma are analogous to those encountered in the treatment of acute lymphoblastic leukemia.

Osteogenic sarcoma

Osteogenic sarcoma is the most common malignant bone tumor of childhood. The prognosis for patients with osteogenic sarcoma has improved markedly in recent decades with the addition of adjuvant and neo-adjuvant chemotherapy to surgical management. High-dose methotrexate has become a standard component of many treatment protocols although an actual correlation between plasma levels of methotrexate and survival is not clear. High-dose methotrexate has been compared to moderate dose methotrexate with conflicting results [48–50]. The current use of high-dose methotrexate in dosages of 8–12 g/m² was pioneered by Rosen et al. in 1978 by escalating the dose of methotrexate in individual patients until a response was achieved [51]. The theoretical advantage of high-dose methotrexate is the biochemical ability to overcome relative methotrexate resistance by administration of a megadose of methotrexate followed by rescue of normal cells by providing reduced folates in the form of leucovorin [reviewed in 25, 52, 53]. With adequate leucovorin rescue and close monitoring of renal function and with vigorous hydration and alkalinization, toxicity secondary to high-dose methotrexate is usually tolerable. The incidence of mucositis, renal failure and myelosuppression is surprisingly low in most studies although unexpected toxicity still occurs [25].

High-dose methotrexate is currently used in combination with other agents known to be active in the treatment of osteogenic sarcoma, notably cisplatin or ifosfamide and adriamycin. The actual contribution of high-dose methotrexate when used in combination with these agents is ambiguous. From a biochemical view, one also needs to be reminded that if the major intracellular target for methotrexate is dihydrofolic acid reductase, then the notion that 'overkill' can be attained is important. As opposed to animal liver and cells grown *in vitro*, human malignant and normal cells have very little dihydrofolic acid reductase. We found that acute lymphoblastic leukemia cells have only 1–5% of the enzyme (expressed as pmoles of methotrexate binding/10^6 cells) found in murine and even human leukemia cells *in vitro* [54]. In eleven adult patients, a dose of only 15 mg methotrexate/m^2 (orally) was found to achieve a methotrexate content in squamous cell carcinomas greater than the DHFR content when measured in biopsy samples the day after the dose [55]. Moreover, at this dose there was more methotrexate in the tumor than in the adjacent normal tissue.

The cost of high-dose methotrexate also cannot be ignored. Use of high-dose methotrexate results in prolonged hospitalization and a need for intensive nursing during chemotherapy administration as well as increased laboratory costs incurred as a result of the necessity of monitoring methotrexate levels.

In summary, although widely accepted as 'standard therapy', it is still our opinion that the role of high-dose methotrexate remains controversial and warrants further investigation [25, 48]. The elimination of high-dose methotrexate except in those patients in whom there is a poor histological response following treatment with other active agents (platinum, adriamycin) needs to be addressed. The omission of high-dose methotrexate would be likely to both decrease the cost of treatment as well as possibly decreasing cumulative toxicity secondary to administration of multiple agents with similar side effects. Of particular concern is renal toxicity when high-dose methotrexate is administered in a regimen that also contains ifosfamide or cisplatin.

Toxicity

Much of the toxicity experienced as a result of the use of methotrexate is similar to that seen after the use of other chemotherapeutic agents. This includes myelosupression, nausea and vomiting and mucositis. Higher doses of methotrexate are associated with nephrotoxicity, probably secondary to intratubular precipitation of methotrexate and/or metabolites. Much of the above toxicity can be managed or prevented with adequate supportive care, close monitoring and judicious use of leucovorin rescue. In particular, high-dose methotrexate requires hydration and alkalinization of the urine in addition to leukovorin.

Methotrexate has also been associated with both acute and chronic hepatotoxicity, the former is typically self-limited and seen with high-dose therapy, the latter is typically associated with chronic use of methotrexate in non-malignant conditions such as psoriasis [56 and reviewed in 2 and 57]. With specific regard to children, it has recently been reported that even the prolonged oral, divided dose methotrexate taken for 30 months in patients with acute lymphoblastic leukemia was commonly associated with increased serum transaminases but, in the absence of hepatitis C, there were no long term sequelae [58].

Pneumonitis has also been described, characterized by fever, cough and interstitial infiltrates [59, 60].

The neurotoxicity of methotrexate is probably of greatest concern because of its unpredictable nature and lack of definitive treatment. There are three well defined syndromes of neurotoxicity secondary to methotrexate. These are 1) an acute syndrome, usually within a day of treatment, manifesting as nausea, emesis, headache, somnolence, lethargy or seizures 2) a subacute syndrome, occurring within one to two weeks after exposure, characterized by seizures, affective disturbances and focal neurological deficits such as transient paresis, blurred vision, aphasia, anesthesia and pseudobulbar palsy and 3) a delayed leukoencephalopathy of variable severity weeks to months following therapy [recently reviewed in 6]. The neurological toxicity of methotrexate is becoming increasingly important, especially in light of the concept of trying to decrease morbidity of therapy in the face of improving survival rates. Although the pathogenesis of methotrexate-induced neurological toxicity is not fully understood, our growing understanding of the biochemical details of folate metabolism offers a unique opportunity for speculation as to the actual events leading to neurological toxicity, as well as for potential clinical intervention to prevent and treat neurological toxicity in patients receiving methotrexate. The effect of methotrexate on adenosine, biopterins and homocysteine with regard to neurotoxicity was recently reviewed [3].

As shown by Cronstein and colleagues [61], accumulation of adenosine is thought to result from accumulation of an intermediate in purine synthesis, 5-aminoimidazole-4-carboxamide ribonucleotide (AICAR), because methotrexate polyglutamates directly inhibit the enzyme. The acute neurotoxic effects of adenosine accumulation seen when patients are given deoxycoformycin (Pentostatin), an inhibitor of adenosine deaminase, have been well described and are similar to those seen with the use of methotrexate [62]. A practical clinical note is that a methylxanthine such as theophylline or caffeine, being an adenosine receptor antagonist, might ameliorate some of the toxicity [63, 64].

Inhibition of the synthesis of neurotransmitters has also been hypothesized as a mechanism of methotrexate toxicity. Biochemical analysis of folate deficient patients revealed decreased plasma concentrations of the major metabolites of dopamine and serotonin [65]. It is possible that methotrexate interferes with neurotransmitter synthesis at the level of biopterin recycling. Potential intervention by pharmacological supplementation with biopterins and neurotransmitters has been reported in one patient with methotrexate neurotoxicity [66, 67].

Lastly, methotrexate interferes with homocysteine metabolism by impairing the regeneration of tetrahydrofolate from dihydrofolate by inhibition of DHFR. That is, methotrexate causes a biochemical deficiency of folate which can then result in a rise in plasma homocysteine. Homocystinemia is associated with vascular disease and damages endothelial cells [68, 69]. Of interest, the endothelial cell damage seen *in vitro* required the addition of exogenous adenosine. The intracellular 'culprit' was s-adenosylhomocysteine (SAH). SAH is a potent inhibitor of methylation reactions. Since application of methotrexate increases both homocysteine and adenosine, the resultant potential for endothelial cell insult may be greater than just seen with a folate deficiency. Increased amounts of homocysteine are also associated with excessive activity of potentially neurotoxic excitatory amino acids which activate the N-methyl D-aspartate (NMDA) receptor [70, reviewed in 3 and 71]. If these biochemical perturbations are responsible for the neurotoxicity then it may be that non-folate analog drugs can provide unique protection for the CNS without use of excess leukovorin. Specifically, dextromethorphan or dextrothorphan are non-competitive antagonists at the NMDA site and betaine can substitute for folate as a methyl donor to convert homocysteine to methionine. This later reaction may or may not take place in the brain, but can certainly decrease plasma homocysteine. The predictive value of this new understanding of neurotoxicity may be as important as the pharmacological intervention. Specifically, a methylenetetrahydrofolate reductase polymorphism is present in about 12% of the population. These patients have mild hyperhomocystinemia. If they are challenged with drugs that cause a folate deficiency, perhaps they are a group of patients likely to have increased neurotoxicity. Further exploration of the role of homocysteine with regard to neurotoxicity, with perhaps even screening of patients prior to administration of methotrexate for hyperhomocystinemia, is warranted.

Conclusion

Folic acid antagonists, primarily methotrexate, have been used for over fifty years, and in spite of many patient years of experience, much is unknown about the administration and metabolism of this commonly used chemotherapeutic agent. With increasing survival of patients with childhood cancer, it is imperative that our current practices be examined critically in a scientific fashion, so as to maximize efficacy and minimize morbidity. The biochemical mechanisms of neurotoxicity should be pursued, especially because of the obvious implications for therapeutic intervention. Lastly, the role of folate metabolism with regard to dietary folate deficiency, excess dietary folate intake and judicious use and overuse of leucovorin needs to be examined.

References

1 Farber S, Diamond L, Mercer R, Sylvester RF, Wolff JA (1948) Temporary remissions in acute leukemia in children produced by folic acid antagonist, 4 amino-pteroyl-glutamic acid (aminopterin). *N Engl J Med* 238: 787–793

2 Bertino JR, Kamen BA (1996) Chemotherapeutic Agents: Folic Acid Antagonists. In: Holland JF, Frei E, Bast RC, Kufe DW, Morton DL, Weichselbaum RR (eds): *Cancer Medicine*. Lea and Febiger, Philadelphia and London, 907–928

3 Crom W (1998) Methotrexate. In: Grochow L, Ames M (eds): *A clinician's guide to chemotherapy pharmacokinetics and pharmacodynamics*. Williams and Wilkins, 311–330

4 Kamen BA (1997) Folate and Antifolate Pharmacology. *Sem Oncol* 24: 18–39

5 Blount BC, Mack MM, Wehr CM, MacGregor JT, Hiatt RA, Wang G, Wickramasinghe SN, Everson RB, Ames BN (1997) Folate deficiency causes uracil mis-incorporation into human DNA and chromosome breakage: Implications for cancer and neuronal damage. *Proc Natl Acad Sci USA* 94: 3290–3295

6 Quinn CT, Kamen BA (1996) A biochemical perspective of methotrexate neurotoxicity with insight on non-folate rescue modalities. *J Invest Med* 44: 522–530

7 Huennekens FM (1994) The methotrexate story: a paradigm for development of cancer therapeutic agents. *Adv Enz Reg* 34: 397–419

8 Smith AS, Hum M, Winick NJ, Kamen BA (1996) A case for the use of aminopterin in treatment of patients with leukemia based upon metabolic studies of blasts *in vitro*. *Clin Cancer Res* 2: 69–73

9 Ratliff AF, Wilson J, Hum M, Marling-Cason M, Rose K, Winick N, Kamen BA (1998) A phase I and pharmacokinetic trial of aminopterin in patients with refractory malignancies. *J Clin Oncol* 16: 1458–1464

10 Zhang L, Taub JW, Williamson M, Wong SC, Hukku B, Pullen J, Ravindranath Y, Matherly LH (1998) Reduced Folate carrier gene expression in childhood acute lymphoblastic leukemia: relationship to immunophenotype and ploidy. *Clin Cancer Res* 4: 2169–2177

11 Egan MG, Sirlin S, Rumberger BG, Garrow TA, Shane B, Sirotnak FM (1995) Rapid decline in folylpolyglutamate synthetase activity and gene expression during maturation of HL-60 cells. *J Biol Chem* 270: 5462–5468

12 Lark RH, Smith AS, Kamen BA (1996) Folylpolyglutamate Synthetase but not folate receptor correlates with MA104 cell growth *in vitro*. *Cancer Res Ther Control* 5: 1–10

13 Weitman SD, Weinberg AG, Coney LR, Zurawski VR, Jennings D, Kamen BA (1992) Cellular localization of the folate receptor: Potential role in drug toxicity and folate homeostasis. *Cancer Res* 52: 6708–6711

14 Weitman S, Anderson RGW, Kamen BA (1994) Folate binding proteins. In: K. Dakshinamurti (ed): *Vitamin receptors: vitamins as ligands in cell communication*. Cambridge. University Press Cambridge, 106–136

15 Gorlick R, Goker E, Trippett T, Steinherz P, Elissesyeff Y, Mazumdar M, Flintoff WF, Bertino JR (1997) Defective transport is a common mechanism of acquired methotrexate resistance in acute lymphocytic leukemia and is associated with decreased reduced folate carrier expression. *Blood* 89: 1013–1018

16 Chazal M, Cheradame S, Formento JL, Francoual M, Formento P, Etienne MC, Francois E, Richelme H, Mousseau M, Letoublon C, et al (1997) Decreased folypolyglutamate synthetase in tumors resistant to fluorouracil-folinic acid treatment: Clinical data. *Clin Cancer Res* 3: 553–557

17 Rhee MS, Wang Y, Nair MG, Galivan J (1993) Acquisition of resistance to antifolates caused by enhanced gamma-glutamyl hydrolase activity. *Cancer Res* 53: 2227–2230

18 Pui C-H, Evans WE (1998) Acute lymphoblastic leukemia. *N Engl J Med* 339: 605–615

19 Simone J (1998) The evolution of cancer care for children and adults. *J Clin Oncol* 16: 2904–2905

20 Law LW (1952) Effects of combinations of antileukemic agents on an acute lymphocytic leukemia of mice. *Cancer Res* 12: 871–878

21 Goldin A, Mantel N, Greenhouse SW, Venditti JM, Humphreys SR (1953) Effect of delayed administration of citrovorum factor on the antileukemic effectiveness of aminopterin in mice. *Cancer Res* 13: 43–48

22 Goldin A, Venditti JM, Humphreys SR, Mantel N Modification of treatment schedules in the management of advanced mouse leukemia with aminopterin. *J Natl Can Inst* 17: 203–212

23 Frei E, Freirech EJ, Gehan E, Pinkel D, Holland JF, Selawry O, Haurani F, Spurr CL, Hayes DM, James W, Rothberg H, et al (1961) Acute leukemia group B, studies of sequential and combination antimetabolite therapy in acute leukemia: 6 mercaptopurine and methotrexate. *Blood* 18: 431–454

24 Jonsson OG, Kamen BA (1991) Methotrexate and Childhood Leukemia. *Cancer Invest* 9: 53–60

25 Ackland SP, Schilsky RL (1987) High-dose methotrexate: A critical reappraisal. *J Clin Oncol* 5: 2017–2031

26 Lange BJ, Blatt J, Sather HN, Meadows AT (1996) Randomized comparison of moderate-dose methotrexate infusions to oral methotrexate in children with intermediate risk acute lymphoblastic leukemia: a children's cancer study group. *Med Pediatr Oncol* 27: 15–20

27 Seidel H, Nygaard R, Moe PJ, Jacobsen G, Lindqvist B, Slørdal L (1997) On the prognostic value of systemic methotrexate clearance in childhood acute lymphoblastic leukemia. *Leukemia Res* 21: 429–434

28 Evans WE, Crom WR, Abromowitch M, Dodge R, Look AT, Bowman WP, George SL, Pui CH (1986) Clinical pharmacodynamics of high-dose methotrexate in acute lymphoblastic leukemia. *N Engl J Med* 314: 471–477

29 Freeman AI, Weinberg V, Brecher ML, et al (1983) Comparison of intermediate dose methotrexate with cranial irradiation for the post-induction treatment of acute lymphocytic leukemia in children. *N Engl J Med* 308: 477–484

30 Abromowitch M, Ochs J, Pui CH, Fairclough D, Murphy SB, Rivera G (1988) Efficacy of high dose methotrexate in childhood acute lymphocytic leukemia: Analysis by contemporary risk classifications. *Blood* 71: 866–869

31 Mahoney DH, Shuster J, Nitschke R, Lauer SJ, Winnick N, Steuber CP, Camitta B (1998) Intermediate – Dose Methotrexate with intravenous mercaptopurine is superior to repetitive low-dose oral methotrexate with intravenous mercaptopurine for children with lower-risk B-lineage acute lymphoblastic leukemia: A Pediatric Oncology Group Phase III Trial. *J Clin Oncol* 16: 246–254

32 Kamen BA, Winnick N, Holcenberg JS (1998) Oral vs. intravenous methotrexate: Another opinion. *J Clin Oncol* 16: 2283–2284

33 Mahoney DH, Shuster JJ, Nitschke R, Lauer SJ, Steuber CP, Winick W, Camitta B (1998) Acute neurotoxicity in children with B-precursor acute lymphoblastic leukemia: an association with intermediate-dose intravenous methotrexate and intrathecal triple therapy – a pediatric oncology group study. *J Clin Oncol* 16: 1712–1722

34 Kamen BA, Vietti T (1989) Oral Leucovorin increases CSF folate concentration in children with leukemia. *Brit J Cancer* 60: 799

35 Nachman JB, Sather HN, Sensel MG, Trigg ME, Cherlow JM, Lukens JN, Wolff L, Uckun FM, Gaynon P (1975) Augmented post-induction therapy for children with high-risk lymphoblastic leukemia and a slow response to initial therapy. *N Engl J Med* 338: 1663–1671

36 Capizzi RL (1975) Improvement in the therapeutic index of methotrexate by l-asparaginase. *Cancer Chem Rep* 6: 37–41

37 Balis FM, Holcenberg JS, Poplack DG, Ge J, Sather HN, Murphy RF, Ames MM, Waskerwitz MJ, Tubergen DG, Zimm S, et al (1998) Pharmacokinetics and pharmacodynamics of oral methotrexate and mercaptopurine in children with lower risk acute lymphoblastic leukemia: A joint Children's Cancer Group and Pediatric Oncology Branch Study. *Blood* 92: 3569–3577

38 Evans WE, Relling MV, Rodman JH, Crom WR, Boyett JM, Pui CH (1998) Conventional compared with individualized chemotherapy for childhood acute lymphoblastic leukemia. *N Engl J Med* 338: 499–505

39 Hum M, Smith A, Lark R, Winick N, Kamen BA (1997) Evidence for negative feedback of extracellular methotrexate (methotrexate) on Acute lymphoblastic leukemia blasts *in vitro*. *Pharmacotherapy* 17: 1260–1266

40 Kamen BA, Holcenberg JS, Turo K, Whitehead VM (1984) Methotrexate and folate content of erythrocytes in patients receiving oral vs. intramuscular therapy with methotrexate. *J Pediatr* 104: 131–133

41 Sansone G (1954) Pathomorphosis of acute infantile leukemia treated with modern therapeutic agents; "meningoleukaemia" and Frolich's obesity. *Annales Paediatrici* 183: 33–42

42 Pinkel D (1979) Treatment of acute lymphocytic leukemia. *Cancer* 43: 1128–1137

43 Pui CH, Mahmoud HM, Rivera G, Hancock ML, Sandlund JT, Behn FG, Head DR, Relling MV, Ribeiro RC, Rubnitz JE, et al (1998) Early intensification of intrathecal chemotherapy virtually eliminates central nervous system relapse in children with acute lymphoblastic leukemia. *Blood* 92: 411–415

44 Balis FM, Lester CM, Chrousos GP, Heideman RL, Poplack DG (1987) Differences in cerebrospinal fluid penetration of corticosteroids: Possible relationship to the prevention of meningeal leukemia. *J Clin Oncol* 5: 202–207

45 Peylan-Ramu N, Poplack DG, Blei CL, et al (1977) Computer assisted tomography in methotrexate encephalopathy. *J Comput Assist Tomogr* 1: 216

46 Wollner N, Burchenal JH, Liebermann PH, Exelby P, D'Angio G, Murphy ML (1976) Non-Hodgkin's Lymphoma in children: a comparative study of two modalities of therapy. *Cancer* 37: 123–134

47 Meadows AT, Sposto R, Jenkin RDT, Kersey JH, Chilcote RR, Siegel SE, Coccia PF, Rosenstock J, Pringle KC, Stolar CJ (1989) Similar efficacy of 6 and 18 months of therapy with four drugs for localized non-Hodgkin's lymphoma of children. A report from the Children's Cancer Study Group. *J Clin Oncol* 7: 92–99

48 Grem JL, King SA, Wittes RE, Jones BL (1988) The role of methotrexate in osteosarcoma. *J Natl Cancer Inst* 80: 626–656

49 Bacci G, Picci P, Ruggieri P, Mercuri M, Avella M, Capanna R, Brach Del Prever A, Mancini A, Gherlinzoni F, Padovani G, et al (1990) Primary Chemotherapy and Delayed Surgery for Osteosarcoma of the extremities. *Cancer* 65: 2539–2553

50 Krailo M, Ertel I, Makley J, Fryer CJH, Baum E, Weetman R, Yunis E, Barnes L, Bleyer WA, Hammond D (1987) A randomized study comparing high-dose methotrexate with moderate dose methotrexate as components of adjuvant chemotherapy in childhood nonmetastatic osteosarcoma: A report form the Childrens Cancer Study Group. *Med Pediatr Oncol* 15: 69–77

51 Rosen G, Huvos AG, Mosende C, Beattie EJ, Exelby PR, Capparos B, Marcove RC (1978) Chemotherapy and thoracotomy for metastatic osteogenic sarcoma: a model for adjuvant chemotherapy and the rational for timing of thoracic surgery. *Cancer* 41: 841–849

52 Kamen BA, Winick NJ (1988) High dose methotrexate: insecure rationale? *Biochem Pharmacol* 37: 2713–2715

53 Bertino JR (1993) Ode to methotrexate. *J Clin Oncol* 11: 5–14

54 Kamen BA, Nylen PA, Whitehead VM, Abelson HT, Dolnick BJ, Peterson DW (1985) Lack of dihydrofolate reductase in human tumor and leukemia cells *in vivo*. *Cancer Drug Delivery* 2: 133–138

55 Schifeling DJ, George T, McGuirt F, Capizzi RL, and Kamen BA (1994) Methotrexate (methotrexate) content in squamous cell carcinoma of the head and neck (SCCHN) after low dose methotrexate. *Med Pediatr Oncol* 22: 88–90

56 Zachariae H, Kragballe K, Sogaard H (1980) Methotrexate induced cirrhosis. *Br J Dermatol* 102: 407–412

57 Kamen BA (1987) Folic acid antagonists. In: Prough RA, Powis G (eds): *Metabolism of Anti-Cancer Drugs*. Taylor and Francis, Ltd, 141–162

58 Farrow AC, Buchanan GR, Zwiener JZ, Bowman WP, Winick NJ (1997) Serum aminotransferase elevation during and following treatment of childhood acute lymphoblastic leukemia. *J Clin Oncol* 15: 1560–1566

59 Sostman HD, Matthay RA, Putnam C, Smith GJ (1976) Methotrexate induced pneumonitis. *Medicine (Baltimore)* 55: 371–388

60 Evans WE, Pratt CB (1978) Effect of pleural effusion on high-dose methotrexate kinetics. *Clin Pharmacol Ther* 23: 68–72

61 Cronstein BN, Eberle MA, Griber HE, Levin RI (1991) Methotrexate inhibits neutrophil function by stimulating adenosine release from connective tissue cells. *Proc Natl Acad Sci USA* 88: 2441–2445

62 Kane BJ, Kuhn JG, Roush MK (1991) Pentostatin: an adenosine deaminase inhibitor for the treatment of hairy cell leukemia. *Ann Pharmacother* 26: 939–947

63 Bernini JC, Fort DW, Griener JC, Kane BJ, Chappell WB, Kamen BA (1995) Aminophylline for methotrexate induced neurotoxicity. *Lancet* 345: 544–547

64 Haider K, Wright J, Lemke S, Gentile T (1998) Reversal of methotrexate induced neurotoxicity by the use of iv aminophylline. First case report in adults. *Blood* 92 suppl: 237a

65 Boetz MI, Young SN, Bachevalier J, Gauthier S (1979) Folate deficiency and decreased brain 5-hydroxytryptamine synthesis in man and rat. *Nature* 278: 182–183

66 Hyland K, Smith I, Bottigleri T, Perry J, Wendel U, Clayton PT, Leonard JV (1988) Demyelination and decreased S-adenosylmethionine in 5,10-methylenetetra-hydrofolate reductase deficiency. *Neurology* 38: 459–462

67 Millot F, Chastagner P, Dhondt J, Sommelet D (1992) Substitutive therapy in a case of methotrexate neurotoxicity. *Eur J Cancer* 28A: 1935

68 Rees MM, Rodgers GM (1993) Homocystinemia: association of a metabolic disorder with vascular disease and thrombosis. *Thromb Res* 71: 337–359

69 Wang H, Yoshizumi M, Lai K, Tsai J-C, Perrella MA, Haber E, Lee ME (1997) Inhibition of growth and p^{21ras} methylation in vascular endothelial cells by homocysteine but not cysteine. *J Biol Chem* 272: 25380–25385

70 Griffiths R (1993) The biochemistry and pharmacology of excitatory sulphur-containing amino acids. *Biochem Soc Trans* 21: 66–72

71 Lipton SA, Rosenberg PA (1994) Excitatory amino acids as a final common pathway for neurologic disorders. *N Engl J Med* 330: 613–622

The mechanisms of methotrexate's action in the treatment of inflammatory disease

Bruce N. Cronstein and Edwin S.L. Chan

New York University School of Medicine, 550 First Ave. New York, NY 10016, USA

Introduction

The introduction of methotrexate for the therapy of rheumatoid arthritis and other forms of inflammatory arthritis has revolutionized the way in which these diseases are now treated. Because methotrexate was introduced empirically for the treatment of inflammatory disease without any specific understanding of a biological basis for its antiinflammatory properties, no improvements on this line of therapy have yet been introduced. A number of recent studies suggest several potential mechanisms of action and new agents developed on the basis of these mechanisms are currently being studied. We will discuss here the biochemical mechanisms by which methotrexate may suppress the inflammation of rheumatoid arthritis.

Methotrexate is a folate antagonist

Methotrexate was originally developed as a specific antagonist of folic acid which, by inhibiting the steps involved in the synthesis of purines and pyrimidines, depletes cellular pools of purines and pyrimidines required for cellular proliferation. Used in the high doses normally employed to treat malignancies this is undoubtedly the mechanism of action of methotrexate, as discussed elsewhere. In contrast, in the treatment of rheumatoid arthritis and other forms of inflammatory arthritis, much lower doses of methotrexate are commonly employed (5–25 mg/week) which probably do not diminish inflammation by inhibiting cellular proliferation. Strong evidence that methotrexate is not acting strictly as a folate antagonist in the treatment of inflammatory arthritis is provided by the widespread and standard practice of administering folic acid or folinic acid with methotrexate for the prevention of undesirable toxicities without reversing the antiinflammatory effects of methotrexate. Further evidence that methotrexate is not simply acting to inhibit cellular proliferation is that methotrexate is usually discontinued, or the dose diminished, if there is significant bone marrow suppression or stomatitis, consequences of diminished cellular proliferation often prevented by folic acid or folinic acid supplementation. Thus, it is likely that there are other biochemical mechanisms responsible for methotrexate's actions in the therapy of inflammatory disease.

Methotrexate inhibits transmethylation reactions

One of the earliest proposals regarding the mechanism of action of methotrexte in the treatment of inflammatory arthritis is the hypothesis that methotrexate inhibits, indirectly, cellular transmethylation reactions. As shown in Figure 1, tetrahydrofolate donates a methyl group to homocysteine forming methionine; methionine can be used in protein synthesis or can be converted to S-adenosylmethionine. S-adenosylmethionine donates a methyl group in a variety of critical intracellular reactions including the methylation of lipids and DNA, and the post-translational modification of proteins and peptides. The S-adenosylhomocysteine that remains after the methylation of cellular target molecules is converted by the action of S-adenosylhomocysteine hydrolase to adenosine, which can be phosphorylated to adenine nucleotides or deaminated to inosine, and homocysteine which can be utilized in protein synthesis or which can then re-enter the cycle to form methionine and S-adenosylmethionine. The transmethylation of cellular lipids and proteins is critical for cellular sur-

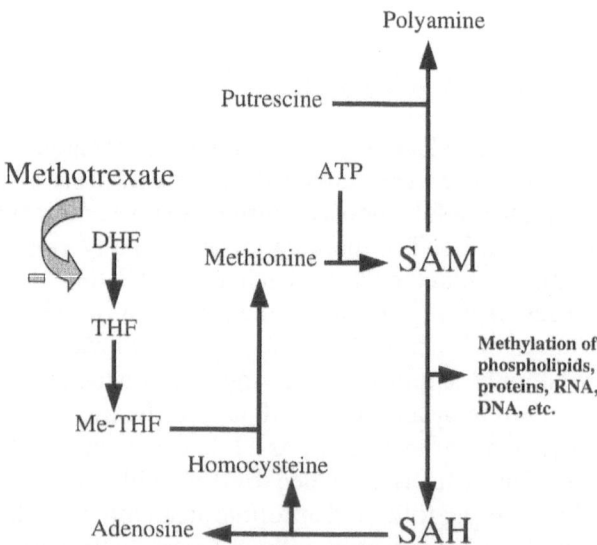

Figure 1. Methotrexate inhibits transmethylation reactions and polyamine formation. DHF = dihydrofolate; THF = tetrahydrofolate; Me-THF = N5-CH$_2$-tetrahydrofolate; ATP = adenosine triphosphate; SAM = S-adenosyl-methionine; SAH = S-adenosyl-homocysteine.

vival although the dependence of specific cell types on transmethylation reactions varies.

Two decades ago it was observed that the red cells and lymphocytes of children suffering from adenosine deaminase deficiency accumulate S-adenosylhomocysteine and the high concentrations of S-adenosyl-homocysteine that accumulate inhibit the formation of S-adenosylmethionine and consequently cellular transmethylation reactions as well [1–4]. That the adenosine deaminase deficiency and the resulting inhibition of cellular transmethylation reactions was associated with a severe combined immunodeficiency suggested that transmethylation reactions might be particularly important in normal immune function. Thus, it was possible that by inhibiting transmethylation reactions the immune response could be blunted in such diseases as rheumatoid arthritis (RA). Evidence for this hypothesis was provided by a series of studies in which inhibition of transmethylation reactions inhibited monocyte and lymphocyte function [5–9]. These observations led to the development of a specific inhibitor of cellular transmethylation reactions, 3-deaza-adenosine, which was an effective inhibitor of immune reactions both *in vitro* and *in vivo*. Because of its success in the pre-clinical studies 3-deaza-adenosine was then administered to patients with rheumatoid arthritis. Despite evidence that the compound did, in fact, inhibit transmethylation reactions in the patients [10] the agent had no beneficial effect on the course of rheumatoid arthritis (M. Weinblatt, personal communication). The experience with this failed therapeutic intervention indicates that it is unlikely that inhibition of transmethylation reactions alone is sufficient to account for the capacity of methotrexate to inhibit inflammation in patients with inflammatory arthritis.

Methotrexate inhibits the formation of polyamines

Inhibition by methotrexate of S-adenosylmethionine formation forms the basis for a second hypothesis accounting for the actions of methotrexate. S-Adenosylmethionine is utilized in the formation of polyamines, such as spermine and spermidine, from putrescine. Polyamines accumulate in the urine, synovial fluid, synovial tissue and monocytes of patients with rheumatoid arthritis. Monocytes and macrophages generate a variety of potentially toxic agents such as NH_3 and H_2O_2 when they metabolize polyamines and these toxic agents have been shown to diminish T lymphocyte interleukin 2 (IL-2) production [11–15]. IL-2 is required for T cell proliferation and the diminished IL-2 production by T cells exposed to the metabolites of these polyamines mirrors the diminished IL-2 production in synovial T cells. Methotrexate, albeit at concentrations greater than those generally achieved in patients treated with low doses of the drug, inhibits the blockage of T cell function *in vitro*. The beneficial effects of methotrexate can be reversed by high concentrations of leukovorin and polyamines. Similarly, the accumulation of polyamines is associated with enhanced B cell formation of rheumatoid factor and altered monocyte function. Methotrexate can reverse these effects. Thus, methotrexate, by inhibiting the accumulation of polyamines, diminishes the production of toxic agents involved in the modulation of T cell, B cell and monocyte function associated with rheumatoid arthritis [11–15]. It should be noted that in patients with rheumatoid arthritis, the synovium is the site for the production of large quantities of toxic oxygen metabolites as a result of the stimulation of various cells by immune reactants (activated complement components and immune complexes among others). Hence, removal of one source of these toxic reactants is probably not sufficient to explain the therapeutic effects of methotrexate. Moreover, it would be expected that 3-deaza-adenosine would interfere with the accumulation of polyamines as well as the transmethylation of lipids, proteins and DNA.

Methotrexate promotes adenosine release

The pharmacological fate of low-dose methotrexate has been well established; methotrexate is present in the serum for a relatively short period of time but is rapidly redistributed to the tissues where it accumulates. In tissues, methotrexate is polyglutamated and remains in the tissues for long periods of time as methotrexate polyglutamates (Fig. 2). Methotrexate polyglutamates are metabolically active with a different spectrum of action than the native compound. Aminoimidazolecarboxamidoribonucleotide (AICAR) transformylase is the enzyme most potently inhibited by the methotrexate polyglutamates that accumulate intracellularly [16, 17]. AICAR transformylase catalyzes the ninth step in the *de novo* synthesis of purines. Evidence that inhibition of AICAR transformylase occurs in the setting of methotrexate is provided by studies in both experimental animals and patients where, both in high doses and doses similar to those used to treat rheumatoid arthritis, AICAR metabolites are present in high concentration in the urine after methotrexate therapy [18, 19]. Moreover, AICAR accumulates in the splenocytes of animals treated with methotrexate at doses similar to those required for the treatment of rheumatoid arthritis [20]. Experiments performed in animals suggested that the intracellular accumulation of AICAR leads to increased concentrations of adenosine, a potent antiinflammatory autacoid, in the extracellular space [20, 21]. The adenosine that accumulates extracellularly results from the dephosphorylation of adenine nucleotides and, ultimately, AMP by ecto-5'nucleotidase [22]. Further studies in animals have demonstrated that the antiinflammatory effects of methotrexate are mediated by adenosine in a model of acute inflammation as well as in the adjuvant arthritis model in the rat [20, 23]. The mechanism by which AICAR promotes release of ade-

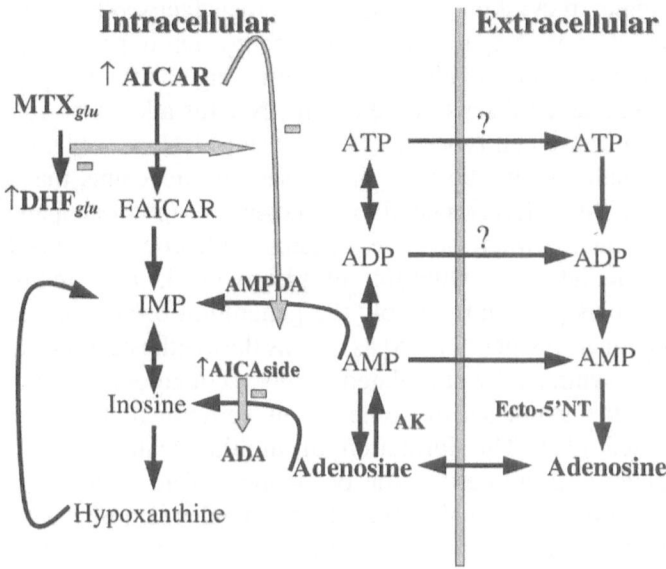

Figure 2. Pathways in adenosine formation. AICAR = 5-aminoimidazole-4-carboxamide ribonucleotide; FAICAR = formyl-AICAR; IMP = inosine monophosphate; AMPDA = AMP deaminase; ADA = adenosine deaminase; AK = adenosine kinase; ecto-5'NT = ecto-5'nucleotidasae.

nine nucleotides remains unclear. The most likely mechanism, at least in part, is through direct inhibition of AMP deaminase activity [24]. Nonetheless, compelling data from animal studies clearly indicates that the mechanism of action of methotrexate is related, at least in part, to an increase in extracellular adenosine generation from AMP in the extracellular fluid [22].

The antiinflammatory effects of adenosine

How does adenosine mediate the antiinflammatory actions of low-dose methotrexate? Adenosine is a ubiquitous autacoid that modulates the function of most tissues and organs via occupancy of specific receptors (recently reviewed in [25]). Currently, there are four known types of adenosine receptors, A_1, A_{2a}, A_{2b}, A_3, that are all members of the large family of seven-transmembrane spanning receptors related to adrenergic receptors. The four adenosine receptors have all been cloned and their sequence is known. The A_1, A_{2a} and A_{2b} receptors are all highly conserved during evolution whereas the A_3 receptor is poorly conserved.

Monocytes and their differentiated tissue forms, macrophages, also play a central role in the pathogenesis of inflammation of rheumatoid arthritis.

The armament of cytokines (e.g. tissue necrosis factor α (TNFα) and IL-1) produced by monocyte/macrophages occupy an important role in the development of acute and chronic inflammation, an effect in part inhibited by methotrexate, as discussed below. mRNA for adenosine receptors are expressed in these cell types (Li M, Cronstein BN, unpublished observation) and methotrexate, through the release of adenosine, may produce a variety of cellular effects related to adenosine receptor occupancy. Adenosine A_1 receptors, when occupied, promote phagocytosis via FcγRI. A_2 receptors mediate the inhibition of phagocytosis of immunoglobulin-coated particles [26] and possibly the generation of superoxide anion by stimulated macrophages [27, 28] as well as the synthesis of nitric oxide and nitric oxide synthase by stimulated monocyte/macrophages [29, 30]. Inhibition of the synthesis of complement component C2 has also been demonstrated [31]. The formation of multinucleated giant cells from macrophages is promoted by the occupancy of adenosine A_1 receptors, which may provide an explanation for the mechanism of the causation of methotrexate-induced nodulosis seen in rheumatoid arthritis [32].

The central role of the neutrophil in inflammation is exemplified by its ubiquitous presence in acute inflammatory infiltrates at the microscopic level. Adenosine exerts its anti-inflammatory effects in part by limiting neutrophil-mediated injury at acutely inflamed sites. Cronstein et al. first demonstrated that adenosine specifically inhibits superoxide anion generation in neutrophils stimulated by the chemoattractant N-formyl-methionyl-leucyl-phenylalanine (fMLP), the complement component C5a, and the calcium ionophore A23187 [33]. This work was further substantiated by studies of adenosine receptor-specific agonists on stimulated oxidant generation, which demonstrated that the adenosine receptor responsible for mediating this function is the A_{2a} receptor [34–36]. The effect of adenosine on stimulated neutrophil degranulation is, however, more controversial. Some laboratories have detected no effect of adenosine on azurophilic granule release [33, 37–39] contrary to observations by others citing an inhibition of stimulated neutrophil degranulation by adenosine [40–42]. Adenosine, acting at adenosine A_1 receptors, also modulates neutrophil chemotaxis [34, 43]. A_1 receptor occupancy also promotes the phagocytosis of immunoglobulin-coated particles [44] and adhesion of neutrophils to endothelial cells and some surfaces [45]. These same functions are however inhibited by the interaction with A_2 receptors [44–46]. Neutrophil adhesion to the vascular endothelium, whether mediated by $\beta2$-integrin or L-selectin, has also been reported to be inhibited by adenosine [45, 47–49]. This inhibition of neutrophil function can be translated to the tissue level where adenosine, whether exogenously added or endogenously generated, has been noted to prevent neutrophil-mediated injury to endothelial cells [50–54]. In contrast to the general effect of adenosine on negating the deleterious functions of the neutrophil in inflammation, Walker et al. reported that adensoine, acting at the A_2 receptor, prevents neutrophils from undergoing apoptosis [55]. The significance of this observation awaits clarification.

In addition to the above described actions of adenosine on neutrophils, monocytes and macrophages, adenosine also promotes granule release from mast cells, an effect mediated by interaction with adenosine A_3 or A_{2b} receptors [56–61]. In the inflamed synovium, methotrexate inhibits the synthesis of collagenase but not tissue inhibitor of metalloprotease (TIMP) or stromelysin in patients with RA, an effect again mediated by adenosine [62, 63]. In endothelial cells, adenosine promotes angiogenesis by inducing endothelial cell migration and proliferation [64, 65]. Along with its effect on the diminution of endothelial expression of E-selectin and intercellular adhesion molecule-1 and secretion of inflammatory cytokines IL-6 and IL-8 [66], adenosine ultimately functions to promote resolution of inflammation and wound healing. Adenosine has also been found to modulate nitric oxide production in the endothelium. Interaction with A_{2a} receptors increase, and interaction with A_1 receptors decrease, the production of nitric oxide by human and porcine arterial endothelial cells [67].

Methotrexate modulates humoral immunity

One of the hallmarks of RA is the presence of antibodies directed against the Fc portion of IgG, rheumatoid factor, in the serum although its role in the pathogenesis of RA is debatable. Several groups have reported that methotrexate treatment does not affect circulating levels of IgM rheumatoid factor [68, 69]. Alarcon and her colleagues [70] studied IgM and IgA rheumatoid factor concentrations in patients involved in a blinded study of the efficacy of methotrexate in the treatment of RA using a sensitive ELISA and observed a significant drop in rheumatoid factor levels in those patients who improved. Analysis of the data showed a strong statistical association between methotrexate treatment and reduction in rheumatoid factor levels and a less impressive association between improvement in response to methotrexate and reduction in rheumatoid factor concentration. Spadaro and colleagues found a reduction in rheumatoid factor levels in RA patients treated with low dose methotrexate [71]. The reduction in IgM rheumatoid factor levels paralleled a decrease in the serum levels of IL-6, and suggested that the action of methotrexate on IgM rheumatoid factor and IL-6 production may stem from a common mechanism [72]. Others have noted that rheumatoid factor levels decreased when inflammation was controlled by either methotrexate or gold salts [73, 74].

Olsen and co-workers reported that treatment of RA patients with methotrexate is associated with diminished rheumatoid factor production by their peripheral blood mononuclear cells cultured *ex vivo* [75] although similar effects on rheumatoid factor production were reported for gold salts as well. Moreover, methotrexate treatment of cultured peripheral blood mononuclear cells leads to diminished rheumatoid factor production *in vitro* [76, 77]. In some of these studies the investigators were able to reverse the effects of methotrexate on rheumatoid factor production by treating the cells with folinic acid.

Since reductions in rheumatoid factor level may accompany successful therapy with other second line agents (e.g. gold salts and penicillamine) and since the role of rheumatoid factor in the pathogenesis of RA is unclear it is difficult to conclude that the effects of methotrexate therapy on rheumatoid factor levels *in vivo* or rheumatoid factor production *in vitro* are causally related to the beneficial effects of this drug in the therapy of RA.

Methotrexate modulates cellular immunity

The central role of cellular immune reactions and T cells in the development and pathogenesis of RA has been generally accepted for a number of years. The strong HLA-DR$_4$-associated risk for development of RA and the presence of large numbers of T cells in the affected synovium support the contention that T cells are important determining elements in the pathogenesis of joint inflammation and destruction in RA. Thus, one potential explanation for the therapeutic effects of methotrexate in RA is diminution in the number or reactivity of T cells involved in the pathogenesis of inflammation in RA, perhaps by inducing apoptosis in activated T cells [78, 79]. In these studies methotrexate promotes apoptosis of antigen-responsive cells by a folate-dependent mechanism. More strikingly, the effects of methotrexate on apoptosis of antigen-stimulated lymphocytes are demonstrable for as long as 24 h after a single dose of the drug [78]. However, it remains difficult to understand how the reversible and temporary induction of apoptosis in T cells can lead to diminished inflammation over prolonged periods of time. Moreover, recent controlled studies of monoclonal antibodies directed against CD4$^+$ T cells have provided little evidence that the elimination or modulation of T cells significantly alters the course of RA [80, 81].

Although a reduction in T cell number or function might be the predicted result of methotrexate treatment, Weinblatt and colleagues [82] reported that, in fact, long-term therapy with methotrexate leads to an increase in the percentage of CD3 and CD4 cells in the peripheral blood. Moreover, those lymphoid cells present in the circulation of patients with RA treated with methotrexate had improved responses to mitogens. In contrast, Wascher et al. reported that short term therapy (12 weeks) diminishes the number of circulating T and B cells [83]. One caveat in interpreting these studies is that peripheral blood T cell number, subsets, or function may not accurately reflect synovial T cell responses. In general, though, there is little data to support the contention that modulation of T cell numbers or functions by methotrexate is responsible for the therapeutic effects of methotrexate.

Methotrexate diminishes phlogiston production and responses

A large and increasing number of soluble agents have been reported to play a role in the development of synovial inflammation. These factors include lipid derivatives (prostaglandins and leukotrienes, platelet activating factor), complement activation products, cytokines and chemokines. Although methotrexate has not been reported to affect the generation of complement activation products or prostaglandins, methotrexate may affect either the generation of or the response to leukotrienes, cytokines and chemokines.

Leukotrienes, most notably leukotriene B_4 (LTB_4), are potent lipid-derived stimuli for leukocytes and the effect of methotrexate therapy on the generation of leukotrienes remains somewhat controversial. Sperling and co-workers have reported that neutrophils from patients or normal controls treated with methotrexate produce less leukotriene B_4 than cells from individuals not treated with methotrexate [84, 85]. Similarly, Leroux and co-workers reported that methotrexate treatment (a single dose) inhibited the generation of 5- and 12-lipoxygenase products [86]. In contrast, Hawkes and her colleagues observed no inhibition by methotrexate administered *in vivo* on the production of lipoxygenase products by neutrophils stimulated *ex vivo* [87]. Methodological differences may account for the differing results. Nonetheless, the resulting diminution in LTB_4 synthesis and synovial fluid concentration is probably not responsible for the therapeutic effects of methotrexate since the magnitude of the decrement in synovial fluid LTB_4 induced by substitution of dietary lipid with fish oil is similar to that induced by methotrexate therapy without leading to as great an improvement in arthritis [88, 89].

Cytokines are low molecular weight proteins which are secreted by various immune and inflammatory cells. Based on studies in animal models of RA, and more recently in patients with RA, it is increasingly clear that cytokines play a critical role in the development of the clinical and laboratory manifestations of RA. Although it is currently thought that tumor necrosis factor α (TNFα) plays a central role in the cytokine cascades responsible for synovial inflammation in RA, IL-1 and IL-6, amongst others, are responsible for many of the manifestations of RA [90]. The effects of methotrexate therapy on both the response to and the production of these cytokines have been studied extensively in animal models, patients and their isolated cells.

IL-1 was among the first cytokines to be discovered. As a result of the availability of reagents with which to measure IL-1 production or the response to IL-1, the levels of this cytokine in both the circulation and synovial fluid of animals and patients with RA has been studied in great detail. In several studies, it has been shown that methotrexate treatment of animals with inflammatory arthritis decreased the production of IL-1 when studied both *in vivo* and *ex vivo* [91–93]. Subsequent studies produced more ambiguous results; methotrexate treatment of either animals, patients or their cells did not inhibit IL-1 production but significantly diminished the ability of their cells to respond to IL-1, an effect which could be overcome in some studies by treatment with folinic acid [94, 95]. One potential explanation for the effects of methotrexate treatment on cellular responses to IL-1 was reported by Brody and colleagues who observed that, when studied *in vitro*, methotrexate markedly inhibited binding of IL-1β to its receptor on peripheral blood cells, an effect that could be overcome by an excess of IL-1β [96]. Although the findings of Brody et al. may explain the *in vitro* effects of methotrexate, it is difficult to understand how reversible inhibition of IL-1 binding can be relevant to the mechanism of action of a drug which is administered on a weekly basis and which is present as free drug in biological fluids for only a matter of hours after the dose is administered [98]. Later studies reported that methotrexate treatment of patients leads to diminished IL-1 concentrations in the synovial fluid of patients who achieved a response to the drug. However, no reduction was observed in their serum IL-1 concentrations [98, 99]. These observations suggested that a local effect of methotrexate treatment on IL-1 production might contribute to the therapeutic effects of low dose methotrexate. Although none of these studies is definitive, they are all consistent with the hypothesis that interference with either IL-1 production or its effects is related to the reduction in symptomatic synovial inflammation observed in patients with RA treated with methotrexate. With the possible exception of the study by Brody et al. [96] none of the studies summarized have determined how methotrexate decreases the secretion of, or the response to, IL-1.

Recently, investigators have focussed their attention on the central role of TNFα in the pathogenesis of RA and this focus has led to the development of potentially useful therapeutic agents (monoclonal anti-TNFα antibodies and soluble TNF receptors). Administration of anti-TNFα antibodies to patients with RA has resulted in dramatic, albeit temporary, improvements in patients with RA (reviewed in [90]). In general, *in vitro* studies of methotrexate using either animal or human cells show that there is little effect of methotrexate on TNFα production although liposomal preparations of methotrexate dramatically inhibit TNFα production *in vitro*, most likely because of improved uptake of liposomal methotrexate by target cells [100–102]. Studies in the adjuvant arthritis model of RA have demonstrated that methotrexate treatment leads to a profound decrease in synovial fluid TNFα concentration [103] and treatment with liposomal methotrexate results in diminished TNFα production *ex vivo* in this model [102]. Neurath et al. in a murine collagen-induced arthritis model, found that intraperitoneal treatment with methotrexate completely prevented the development of arthritis, associated with a striking reduction in splenic TNFα production [104]. Similar reductions in TNFα expression were observed on synovial tissue during methotrexate treatment of synovial biopsies from RA patients in a study by Dolhain and colleagues, where concomitant decreases in IL-1β and adhesion molecules E-selectin and VCAM-1 have also been noted [105]. The studies reported to date do not demonstrate any significant effect of methotrexate therapy on TNFα concentrations in peripheral blood in patients with RA [106]. As with IL-1 (*vide supra*) there may be a disparity between the effects of methotrexate on synovial production of TNFα and total circulating TNFα and the utility of measuring circulating TNFα concentrations as an indicator of response to therapy remains unclear. Thus, although methotrexate therapy leads to a decrease in TNFα production locally, the role of this reduction in the mechanism of action of methotrexate is not settled.

A variety of other pro- and anti-inflammatory proteins have been measured in the serum of RA patients treated with methotrexate. Of these the one cytokine most consistently diminished in the serum is IL-6, a cytokine most tightly linked to production of acute phase reactants by the liver. Serum concentrations of IL-6 declined after methotrexate therapy in association with improved clinical parameters in three studies [72, 107, 108] but did not change in others [109]. Although methotrexate therapy leads to an increase in cellular production of IL-1 receptor antagonist and soluble TNF receptors [110] these changes are not reflected by alterations in circulating levels of these anti-inflammatory proteins. The chemokine IL-8 is a potent chemoattractant for neutrophils and an angiogenic factor produced by mononuclear cells, among others. In patients with RA, methotrexate therapy inhibited spontaneous Il-8 production by peripheral blood mononuclear cells but not synoviocytes from patients with RA [110, 111]. As with the other cytokines studied, the mechanistic role of IL-8 inhibition by methotrexate therapy in the antiinflammatory effects of methotrexate remains uncertain. Constantin and his co-workers reported that *ex vivo* methotrexate treatment of peripheral blood mononuclear cells of RA patients increased IL-4 and IL-10 gene expression and consequently cytokine production while that of IL-2 and interferon-γ were found to be significantly decreased [112]. These results suggested that methotrexate's phlogistic actions may exert a net effect by increasing Th2 cytokines and decreasing Th1 cytokines, compatible with its anti-inflammatory and immunoregulatory actions seen *in vivo*.

The studies summarized above suggest that at least one of the mechanisms by which methotrexate inhibits inflammation in RA is to modulate the production of cytokines in the synovium of patients with RA. Although the production of some of these factors was clearly inhibited by methotrexate treatment *in vitro* or *ex vivo*, other agents also affected cytokine release (e.g. corticosteroids) indicating that the diminution of cytokine release at inflamed sites is not a specific property of methotrexate. Finally, none of the studies cited addressed the question of the molecular mechanism by which methotrexate treatment modulates cytokine release although a number of hypotheses have been suggested.

From benchside to bedside

Methotrexate has been widely used in clinical practice in diseases as diverse as rheumatoid arthritis, psoriasis and asthma. The mechanisms of action of methotrexate discussed above provide insights into the therapeutic modification of disease processes which forms the basis of the clinical efficacy as well as some well documented side effects of methotrexate treatment as applied to these diseases. Inflammatory diseases, in general, require the participation of a host of inflammatory cells such as neutrophils, monocytes/macrophages, lymphocytes, etc. in mediating tissue damage. Inhibition of the synthesis of complement component C2, neutrophil adhesion and superoxide anion generation all contribute to the ability of methotrexate to limit tissue destruction at the inflammatory site through adenosine release. On the other hand, these actions as well as the phagocytosis of immunoglobulin-coated particles, all limited by methotrexate, are important means by which we defend ourselves from microbial invasion, as reflected in the increased incidence of infection during methotrexate therapy. The fusion of macrophages in tissues, again mediated by adenosine, results in the formation of multinucleated giant cells and consequently, granulomata, such as those seen in the cutaneous nodulosis arising from methotrexate therapy [113]. Methotrexate induces apoptosis in keratinocytes and inhibits their proliferation, and these actions have found clinical application in resistant psoriasis [114, 115]. Adenosine release may also account for hepatic fibrosis such as that seen in methotrexate therapy, a subject currently under investigation.

Conclusion

Our knowledge of anti-inflammatory drugs in the treatment of rheumatic disease is impoverished by a lack of thorough understanding of their mechanisms of anti-inflammatory action. Interest in methotrexate and, in particular, its cellular actions mediated through adenosine release in recent years has brought new understanding to these issues. It is our hope that this new and growing wisdom may find its appurtenant role in the creation of new drugs in the advancement of anti-inflammatory therapy.

References

1 Hershfield MS, Kredich NM, Ownby DR, Ownby H, Buckley R (1979) *In vivo* inactivation of erythrocyte S-adenosylhomocysteine hydrolase by 2'-deoxyadenosine in adenosine deaminase-deficient patients. *J Clin Invest* 63: 807–811
2 Kredich NM, Hershfield MS (1979) S-Adenosylhomocysteine toxicity in normal and adenosine kinase-deficient lymphoblasts of human origin. *Proc Natl Acad Sci (USA)* 76: 2450–2455
3 Hershfield MS, Kurtzberg J, Aiyar VN, Suh EJ, Schiff R (1985) Abnormalities in S-adenosylhomocysteine hydrolysis, ATP catabolism, and lymphoid differentiation in adenosine deaminase deficiency. *Ann NY Acad Sci* 451: 78–86

4 Hershfield MS, Krodich NM (1978) S-adenosylhomocysteine hydrolase is an adenosine-binding protein: a target for adenosine toxicity. *Science* 202: 757–760

5 Jurgensen CH, Wolberg G, Zimmerman TP (1989) Inhibition of neutrophil adherence to endothelial cells by 3- deazaadenosine. *Agents Actions* 27: 398–400

6 Jurgensen CH, Huber BE, Zimmerman TP, Wolberg G (1990) 3-deazaadenosine inhibits leukocyte adhesion and ICAM-1 biosynthesis in tumor necrosis factor-stimulated human endothelial cells. *J Immunol* 144: 653–661

7 Prus KL, Wolberg G, Keller PM, Fyfe JA, Stopford CR, Zimmerman TP (1989) 3-deazaadenosine 5'-triphosphate: a novel metabolite of 3- deazaadenosine in mouse leukocytes. *Bio Pharmacol* 38: 509–517

8 Stopford CR, Wolberg G, Prus KL, Reynolds-Vaughn R, Zimmerman TP (1985) 3-deazaadenosine-induced disorganization of macrophage microfilaments. *Proc Natl Acad Sci (USA)* 82: 4060–4064

9 Zimmerman TP, Wolberg G, Duncan GS (1978) Inhibition of lymphocyte-mediated cytolysis by 3-deazaadenosine: evidence for a methylation reaction essential for cytolysis. *Proc Natl Acad Sci (USA)* 75: 6220–6224

10 Smith DM, Johnson JA, Turner RA (1991) Biochemical perturbations of BW 91Y (3-deazaadenosine) on human neutrophil chemotactic potential and lipid metabolism. *Int J Tiss React* 13: 1–18

11 Flescher E, Bowlin TL, Ballester A, Houk R, Talal N (1989) Increased polyamines may downregulate interleukin 2 production in rheumatoid arthritis. *J Clin Invest* 83: 1356–1362

12 Flescher E, Bowlin TL, Talal N (1992) Regulation of IL-2 production by mononuclear cells from rheumatoid arthritis synovial fluids. *Clin Exp Imm* 87: 435–437

13 Nesher G, Moore TL (1990) The *in vitro* effects of methotrexate on peripheral blood mononuclear cells. Modulation by methyl donors and spermidine. *Arthritis Rheum* 33: 954–959

14 Yukioka K, Wakitani S, Yukioka M, Furumitsu Y, Shichikawa K, Ochi T, Goto H, Matsui-Yuasa I, Otani S, Nishizawa Y, et al (1992) Polyamine levels in synovial tissues and synovial fluids of patients with rheumatoid arthritis. *J Rheum* 19: 689–692

15 Talal N, Tovar Z, Dauphinee MJ, Flescher E, Dang H, Galarza D (1988) Abnormalities of T cell activation in the rheumatoid synovium detected with monoclonal antibodies to CD3. *Scand J Rheum – Supplement* 76: 175–182

16 Allegra CJ, Drake JC, Jolivet J, Chabner BA (1985) Inhibition of phosphoribosylaminoimidazolecarboxamide transformylase by methotrexate and dihydrofolic acid polyglutamates. *Proc Natl Acad Sci (USA)* 82: 4881–4885

17 Chabner BA, Allegra CJ, Curt GA, Clendeninn NJ, Baram J, Koizumi S, Drake JC, Jolivet J (1985) Polyglutamation of methotrexate. Is methotrexate a prodrug? *J Clin Invest* 76: 907–912

18 Baggott JE, Morgan SL, Koopman WJ (1998) The effect of methotrexate and 7-hydroxymethotrexate on rat adjuvant arthritis and on urinary aminoimidazole carboxamide excretion. *Arthritis Rheum* 41: 1407–1410

19 Luhby AL, Cooperman JH (1962) Aminoimidazole carboxamide excretion in vitamin B12 and folic acid deficiencies. *Lancet* 2: 1381–1382

20 Cronstein BN, Naime D, Ostad E (1993) The antiinflammatory mechanism of methotrexate: increased adenosine release at inflamed sites diminishes leukocyte accumulation in an *in vivo* model of inflammation. *J Clin Invest* 92: 2675–2682

21 Gruber HE, Hoffer ME, McAllister DR, Laikind PK, Lane TA, Schmid-Schoenbein GW, Engler RL (1989) Increased adenosine concentration in blood from ischemic myocardium by AICA riboside: effects on flow, granulocytes and injury. *Circulation* 80: 1400–1411

22 Morabito L, Montesinos MC, Schreibman DM, Balter L, Thompson LF, Resta R, Carlin G, Huie MA, Cronstein BN (1998) Methotrexate and sulfasalazine promote adenosine release by a mechanism that requires ecto-5'-nucleotidase-mediated conversion of adenine nucleotides. *J Clin Invest* 101: 295–300

23 Montesinos MC, Yap IS, Desai A, Posadas I, McCrary CT, Cronstein BN (2000) Reversal of the antiinflammatory effects of methotrexate by the nonselective adenosine receptor antagonist theophylline and caffeine. *Arthritis Rheum* 43: 656–663

24 Baggott JE, Vaughn WH, Hudson BB (1986) Inhibition of 5-aminoimidazole-4-carboxamide ribotide transformylase, adenosine deaminase and 5'-adenylate deaminase by poly-

glutamates of methotrexate and oxidized folates and by 5-aminoimidazole-4-carboxamide riboside and ribotide. *Biochem J* 236: 193–200

25 Poulsen SA, Quinn RJ (1998) Adenosine receptors: new opportunities for future drugs. *Bioorg Med Chem* 6: 619–641

26 Salmon JE, Brogle N, Brownlie C, Edberg JC, Chen B-X, Erlanger BF (1993) Human mononuclear phagocytes express adenosine A1 receptors: a novel mechanism for differential regulation of Fc-gamma receptor function. *J Immunol* 151: 2775–2785

27 Elliott KRF, Stevenson HC, Miller PJ, Leonard EJ (1986) Synergistic action of adenosine and Fmet-leu-phe in raising cyclic AMP content of purified human monocytes. *Biochem Biophys Res Comm* 138: 1376–1382

28 Leonard EJ, Shenai A, Skeel A (1987) Dynamics of chemotactic peptide-induced superoxide generation by human monocytes. *Inflammation* 11: 229–240

29 Hasko G, Szabo C, Nemeth ZH, Kvetan V, Pastores SM, Vizi ES (1996) Adenosine receptor agonists differentially regulate IL-10, TNF-alpha, and nitric oxide production in RAW 264.7 macrophages and in endotoxemic mice. *J Immunol* 157: 4634–4640

30 Hon WM, Moochhala S, Khoo HE (1997) Adenosine and its receptor agonists potentiate nitric oxide synthase expression induced by lipopolysaccharide in RAW 264.7 murine macrophages. *Life Sciences* 60: 1327–1335

31 Lappin D, Whaley K (1984) Adenosine A2 receptors on human monocytes modulate C2 production. *Clin Exp Immunol* 57: 454–460

32 Merrill JT, Coffey D, Shen C, Zakharenko O, Zhang HW, Lahita RG, Cronstein BN (1995) Mechanisms of rheumatoid nodulosis: methotrexate-enhanced monocyte fusion requires protein synthesis and intact microtubules. *Arth Rheum* 38 (Suppl): S157

33 Cronstein BN, Kramer SB, Weissmann G, Hirschhorn R (1983) Adenosine: a physiological modulator of superoxide anion generation by human neutrophils. *J Exp Med* 158: 1160–1177

34 Cronstein BN, Duguma L, Nicholls D, Hutchison A, Williams M (1990) The adenosine/neutrophil paradox resolved. Human neutrophils possess both A1 and A2 receptors which promote chemotaxis and inhibit O_2-generation, respectively. *J Clin Invest* 85: 1150–1157

35 van Calker D, Steber R, Klotz KN, Greil W (1991) Carbamazepine distinguishes between adenosine receptors that mediate different second messenger responses. *Eur J Pharmacol* 206: 285–290

36 Fredholm BB, Zhang Y, van der Ploeg I (1996) Adenosine A2A receptors mediate the inhibitory effect of adenosine on formyl-Met-Leu-Phe-stimulated respiratory burst in neutrophil leucocytes. *Naunyn-Schmiedebergs Archiv Pharmacol* 354: 262–267

37 Marone G, Thomas L, Lichtenstein L (1980) The role of agonists that activate adenylate cyclase in the control of cAMP metabolism and enzyme release by human polymorphonuclear leukocytes. *J Immunol* 125: 2277–2283

38 McGarrity ST, Stephenson AH, Webster RO (1989) Regulation of human neutrophil functions by adenine nucleotides. *J Immunol* 142: 1986–1994

39 Cronstein BN, Kramer SB, Rosenstein ED, Korchak HM, Weissmann G, Hirschhorn R (1988) Occupancy of adenosine receptors raises cyclic AMP alone and in synergy with occupancy of chemoattractant receptors and inhibits membrane depolarization. *Biochem J* 252: 709–715

40 Bouma MG, Jeunhomme TMMA, Boyle DL, Dentener MA, Voitenok NN, van den Wildenberg FAJM, Buurman WA (1997) Adenosine inhibits neutrophil degranulation in activated human whole blood; involvement of adenosine A2 and A3 receptors. *J Immunol* 158: 5400–5408

41 Richter J (1992) Effect of adenosine analogues and cAMP-raising agents on TNF-, GM-CSF-, and chemotactic peptide-induced degranulation in single adherent neutrophils. *J Leukocyte Biol* 51: 270–275

42 Schmeichel CJ, Thomas LL (1987) Methylxanthine bronchodilators potentiate multiple human neutrophil functions. *J Immunol* 138: 1896–1903

43 Rose FR, Hirschhorn R, Weissmann G, Cronstein BN (1988) Adenosine promotes neutrophil chemotaxis. *J Exp Med* 167: 1186–1194

44 Salmon JE, Cronstein BN (1990) Fcgamma Receptor-Mediated functions in neutrophils are modulated by adenosine receptor occupancy: A1 receptors are stimulatory and A2 receptors are inhibitory. *J Immunol* 145: 2235–2240

45 Cronstein BN, Levin RI, Philips MR, Hirschhorn R, Abramson SB, Weissmann G (1992) Neutrophil adherence to endothelium is enhanced via adenosine A1 receptors and inhibited via adenosine A2 receptors. *J Immunol* 148: 2201–2206

46 Zalavary S, Stendahl O, Bengtsson T (1994) The role of cyclic AMP, calcium and filamentous actin in adenosine modulation of Fc receptor-mediated phagocytosis in human neutrophils. *Biochim Biophys Acta* 1222: 249–256

47 Firestein GS, Bullough DA, Erion MD, Jimenez R, Ramirez-Weinhouse M, Barankiewicz J, Smith CW, Gruber HE, Mullane KM (1995) Inhibition of neutrophil adhesion by adenosine and an adenosine kinase inhibitor: the role of selectins. *J Immunol* 154: 326–334

48 Wollner A, Wollner S, Smith JB (1993) Acting via A2 receptors, adenosine inhibits the upregulation of Mac-1 (CD11b/CD18) expression on FMLP-stimulated neutrophils. *Am J Resp Cell Mol Biol* 9: 179–185

49 Thiel M, Chambers JD, Chouker A, Fischer S, Zourelidis C, Bardenheuer HJ, Arfors KE, Peter K (1996) Effect of adenosine on the expression of beta(2) integrins and L-selectin of human polymorphonuclear leukocytes *in vitro*. *J Leuko Biol* 59: 671–682

50 Cronstein BN, Levin RI, Belanoff J, Weissmann G, Hirschhorn R (1986) Adenosine: an endogenous inhibitor of neutrophil-mediated injury to endothelial cells. *J Clin Invest* 78: 760–770

51 Boisseau MR, Pruvost A, Renard M, Closse C, Belloc F, Seigneur M, Maurel A (1996) Effect of buflomedil on the neutrophil-endothelial cell interaction under inflammatory and hypoxia conditions. *Haemostasis* 26: 182–188

52 Zhao ZQ, Sato H, Williams MW, Fernandez AZ, Vinten-Johansen J (1996) Adenosine A2-receptor activation inhibits neutrophil-mediated injury to coronary endothelium. *Amer J Physiol* 271: H1456–1464

53 Minamino T, Kitakaze M, Node K, Funaya H, Inoue M, Hori M, Kamada T (1996) Adenosine inhibits leukocyte-induced vasoconstriction. *Amer J Physiol* 271: H2622–2628

54 Jordan JE, Zhao ZQ, Sato H, Taft S, Vinten-Johansen J (1997) Adenosine A2 receptor activation attenuates reperfusion injury by inhibiting neutrophil accumulation, superoxide generation and coronary endothelial adherence. *J Pharmacol Exp Therapeutics* 280: 301–309

55 Walker BA, Rocchini C, Boone RH, Ip S, Jacobson MA (1997) Adenosine A2a receptor activation delays apoptosis in human neutrophils. *J Immunol* 158: 2926–2931

56 Feoktistov I, Biaggioni I (1995) Adenosine A2b receptors evoke interleukin-8 secretion in human mast cells An enprofylline-sensitive mechanism with implications for asthma. *J Clin Invest* 96: 1979–1986

57 Hannon JP, Pfannkuche HJ, Fozard JR (1995) A role for mast cells in adenosine A3 receptor-mediated hypotension in the rat. *Br J Pharmacol* 115: 945–952

58 Ali H, Choi OH, Fraundorfer PF, Yamada K, Gonzaga HM, Beaven MA (1996) Sustained activation of phospholipase D via adenosine A3 receptors is associated with enhancement of antigen- and Ca(2+)-ionophore-induced secretion in a rat mast cell line. *J Pharmacol Exp Therapeutics* 276: 837–845

59 Fozard JR, Pfannkuche HJ, Schuurman HJ (1996) Mast cell degranulation following adenosine A3 receptor activation in rats. *Eur J Pharmacol* 298: 293–297

60 Shepherd RK, Linden J, Duling BR (1996) Adenosine-induced vasoconstriction *in vivo* Role of the mast cell and A3 adenosine receptor. *Circ Res* 78: 627–634

61 Meade CJ, Mierau J, Leon I, Ensinger HA (1996) *In vivo* role of the adenosine A3 receptor: N6-2-(4-aminophenyl)ethyladenosine induces bronchospasm in BDE rats by a neurally mediated mechanism involving cells resembling mast cells. *J Pharmacol Exp Therapeutics* 279: 1148–1156

62 Firestein GS, Paine MM, Boyle DL (1994) Mechanisms of methotrexate action in rheumatoid arthritis. Selective decrease in synovial collagenase gene expression. *Arth Rheum* 37: 193–200

63 Boyle DL, Sajjadi FG, Firestein GS (1996) Inhibition of synoviocyte collagenase gene expression by adenosine receptor stimulation. *Arth Rheum* 39: 923–930

64 Sexl V, Mancusi G, Baumgartner-Parzer S, Schutz W, Freissmuth M (1995) Stimulation of human umbilical vein endothelial cell proliferation by A2-adenosine and beta 2-adrenoceptors. *Br J Pharmacol* 114: 1577–1586

65 Ethier MF, Chander V, Dobson JG Jr (1993) Adenosine stimulates proliferation of human endothelial cells in culture. *Amer J Physiol* 265: H131–H138

66 Bouma MG, van den Wildenberg FAJM, Buurman WA (1996) Adenosine inhibits cytokine release and expression of adhesion molecules by activated human endothelial cells. *Amer J Physiol* 39: C522–C529

67 Li J, Fenton RA, Wheeler HB, Powell CC, Peyton BD, Cutler BS, Dobson JG, Jr (1998) Adenosine A2a receptors increase arterial endothelial cell nitric oxide. *J Surg Res* 80: 357–364

68 Singh Y, Sharma M, Singh RR, Kumar A, Malaviya R, Malaviya AN (1992) Methotrexate: clinical and immunological effects in refractory rheumatoid arthritis. *J Assoc Physicians India* 40: 658–661

69 Drosos AA, Psychos D, Andonopoulos AP, Stefanaki-Nikou S, Tsianos EB, Moutsopoulos HM (1990) Methotrexate therapy in rheumatoid arthritis. A two year prospective follow-up. *Clin Rheumatol* 9: 333–341

70 Alarcon GS, Schrohenloher RE, Bartolucci AA, Ward JR, Williams HJ, Koopman WJ (1990) Suppression of rheumatoid factor production by methotrexate in patients with rheumatoid arthritis. Evidence for differential influences of therapy and clinical status on IgM and IgA rheumatoid factor expression. *Arth Rheum* 33: 1156–1161

71 Spadaro A, Riccieri V, Sili Scavalli A, Taccari E, Zoppini A (1993) One year treatment with low dose methotrexate in rheumatoid arthritis: effect on class specific rheumatoid factors. *Clin Rheumatol* 12: 357–360

72 Spadaro A, Taccari E, Riccieri V, Sensi F, Sili Scavalli A, Zoppini A (1997) Relationship of soluble interleukin-2-receptor and interleukin-6 with class-specific rheumatoid factors during low-dose methotrexate treatment in rheumatoid arthritis. *Rev Rheum Engl Ed* 64: 89–94

73 Olsen NJ, Teal GP, Brooks RH (1991) IgM-rheumatoid factor and responses to second-line drugs in rheumatoid arthritis. *Agents Actions* 34: 169–171

74 Moore S, Ruska K, Peters L, Olsen NJ (1994) Associations of IgA and IgA-rheumatoid factor with disease features in patients with rheumatoid arthritis. *Immunol Invest* 23: 355–365

75 Olsen NJ, Callahan LF, Pincus T (1987) Immunologic studies of rheumatoid arthritis patients treated with methotrexate. *Arth Rheum* 30: 481–488

76 Nesher G, Moore TM (1990) The *in vitro* effects of methotrexate on peripheral blood mononuclear cells: modulation by methyl donors and spermidine. *Arth Rheum* 33: 954–959

77 Olsen NJ, Murray LM (1989) Antiproliferative effects of methotrexate on peripheral blood mononuclear cells. *Arth Rheum* 32: 378–385

78 Genestier L, Paillot R, Fournel S, Ferraro C, Miossec P, Revillard JP (1998) Immunosuppressive properties of methotrexate: apoptosis and clonal deletion of activated peripheral T cells. *J Clin Invest* 102: 322–328

79 Segal R, Mozes E, Yaron M, Tartakovsky B (1989) The effects of methotrexate on the production and activity of interleukin-1. *Arth Rheum* 32: 370–377

80 Moreland LW, Pratt PW, Mayes MD, Postlethwaite A, Weisman MH, Schnitzer T, Lightfoot R, Calabrese L, Zelinger DJ, Woody JN, et al (1995) Double-blind, placebo-controlled multicenter trial using chimeric monoclonal anti-CD4 antibody, cM-T412, in rheumatoid arthritis patients receiving concomitant methotrexate. *Arth Rheum* 38: 1581–1588

81 van der Lubbe PA, Dijkmans BA, Markusse HM, Nassander U, Breedveld FC (1995) A randomized, double-blind, placebo-controlled study of CD4 monoclonal antibody therapy in early rheumatoid arthritis. *Arth Rheum* 38: 1097–1106

82 Weinblatt ME, Trentham DE, Fraser PA, Holdsworth DE, Falchuk KR, Weissman BN, Coblyn JS (1988) Long-term prospective trial of low-dose methotrexate in rheumatoid arthritis. *Arth Rheum* 31: 167–175

83 Wascher TC, Hermann J, Brezinschek HP, Brezinschek R, Wilders-Truschnig M, Rainer F, Krejs GJ (1994) Cell-type specific response of peripheral blood lymphocytes to methotrexate in the treatment of rheumatoid arthritis. *Clin Invest* 72: 535–540

84 Sperling RI, Coblyn JS, Larkin JK, Benincaso AI, Austen KF, Weinblatt ME (1990) Inhibition of leukotriene B_4 synthesis in neutrophils from patients with rheumatoid arthritis by a single oral dose of methotrexate. *Arth Rheum* 33: 1149–1155

85 Sperling RI, Benincaso AI, Anderson RJ, Coblyn JS, Austen KF, Weinblatt ME (1992) Acute and chronic suppression of leukotriene B_4 synthesis *ex vivo* in neutrophils from patients with rheumatoid arthritis beginning treatment with methotrexate. *Arth Rheum* 35: 376–384

86 Leroux JL, Damon M, Chavis C, Paulet A rastes de, Blotman F (1992) Effects of a single dose of methotrexate on 5- and 12-lipoxygenase products in patients with rheumatoid arthritis. *J Rheum* 19: 863–866

87 Hawkes JS, Cleland LG, Proudman SM, James MJ (1994) The effect of methotrexate on *ex vivo* lipoxygenase metabolism in neutrophils from patients with rheumatoid arthritis. *J Rheum* 21: 55–58

88 Kremer JM, Jubiz W, Michalek A, Rynes RI, Bartholomew LE, Bigaouette J, Timchalk M, Beeler D, Lininger L (1987) Fish-oil fatty acid supplementation in active rheumatoid arthritis. A double-blinded, controlled, crossover study. *Ann Intern Med* 106: 497–503

89 Kremer JM, Lawrence DA, Jubiz W, DiGiacomo R, Rynes R, Bartholomew LE, Sherman M (1990) Dietary fish oil and olive oil supplementation in patients with rheumatoid arthritis. Clinical and immunologic effects. *Arth Rheum* 33: 810–820

90 Maini RN, Elliott MJ, Brennan FM, Williams RO, Chu CQ, Paleolog E, Charles PJ, Taylor PC, Feldmann M (1995) Monoclonal anti-TNF alpha antibody as a probe of pathogenesis and therapy of rheumatoid disease. [Review]. *Immunol Rev* 144: 195–223

91 Johnson WJ, DiMartino MJ, Meunier PC, Muirhead KA, Hanna N (1988) Methotrexate inhibits macrophage activation as well as vascular and cellular inflammatory events in rat adjuvant induced arthritis. *J Rheumatol* 15: 745–749

92 DiMartino MJ, Johnson WJ, Votta B, Hanna N (1987) Effect of antiarthritic drugs on the enhanced interleukin-1 (IL-1) production by macrophages from adjuvant-induced arthritic (AA) rats. *Agents Actions* 21: 348–350

93 Novaes GS, Mello SB, Laurindo IM, Cossermelli W (1996) Low dose methotrexate decreases intraarticular prostaglandin and interleukin 1 levels in antigen induced arthritis in rabbits. *J Rheumatol* 23: 2092–2097

94 Segal R, Mozes E, Yaron M, Tartakovsky B (1989) The effects of methotrexate on the production and activity of interleukin-1. *Arth Rheum* 32: 370–377

95 Chang DM, Baptiste P, Schur PH (1990) The effect of antirheumatic drugs on interleukin 1 (IL-1) activity and IL-1 and IL-1 inhibitor production by human monocytes. *J Rheumatol* 17: 1148–1157

96 Brody M, Bohm I, Bauer R (1993) Mechanism of action of methotrexate: experimental evidence that methotrexate blocks the binding of interleukin 1 beta to the interleukin 1 receptor on target cells. *Eur J Clin Chem Clin Biochem* 31: 667–674

97 Tishler M, Caspi D, Graff E, Segal R, Peretz H, Yaron M (1989) Synovial and serum levels of methotrexate during methotrexate therapy of rheumatoid arthritis. *Br J Rheumatol* 28: 422–423

98 Chang DM, Weinblatt ME, Schur PH (1992) The effects of methotrexate on interleukin 1 in patients with rheumatoid arthritis. *J Rheumatol* 19: 1678–1682

99 Bondeson J (1997) The mechanisms of action of disease-modifying antirheumatic drugs: a review with emphasis on macrophage signal transduction and the induction of pro-inflammatory cytokines. *Gen Pharmacol* 29: 127–150

100 Williams AS, Punn YL, Amos N, Cooper AM, Williams BD (1995) The effect of liposomally conjugated methotrexate upon mediator release from human peripheral blood monocytes. *Br J Rheumatol* 34: 241–245

101 Williams AS, Topley N, Williams BD (1994) Effect of liposomally encapsulated MTX-DMPE conjugates upon TNF alpha and PGE2 release by lipopolysaccharide stimulated rat peritoneal macrophages. *Biochim Biophys Acta* 1225: 217–222

102 Williams AS, Camilleri JP, Topley N, Williams BD (1994) Prostaglandin and tumor necrosis factor secretion by peritoneal macrophages isolated from normal and arthritic rats treated with liposomal methotrexate. *J Pharmacol Toxicol Methods* 32: 53–58

103 Smith-Oliver T, Noel LS, Stimpson SS, Yarnall DP, Connolly KM (1993) Elevated levels of TNF in the joints of adjuvant arthritic rats. *Cytokine* 5: 298–304

104 Neurath MF, Hildner K, Becker C, Schlaak JF, Barbulescu K, Germann T, Schmitt E, Schirmacher P, Haralambous S, Pasparakis M, et al (1999) Methotrexate specifically modulates cytokine production by T cells and macrophages in murine collagen-induced arthritis (CIA): a mechanism for methotrexate-mediated immunosuppression. *Clin Exp Immunol* 115: 42–55

105 Dolhain RJ, Tak PP, Dijkmans BA, De Kuiper P, Breedveld FC, Miltenburg AM (1998) Methotrexate reduces inflammatory cell numbers, expression of monokines and of ad-

hesion molecules in synovial tissue of patients with rheumatoid arthritis. *Br J Rheumatol* 37: 502–508

106 Barrera P, Boerbooms AM, Janssen EM, Sauerwein RW, Gallati H, Mulder J, de Boo T, Demacker PN, van de Putte LB, van der Meer JW (1993) Circulating soluble tumor necrosis factor receptors, interleukin-2 receptors, tumor necrosis factor alpha, and interleukin-6 levels in rheumatoid arthritis. Longitudinal evaluation during methotrexate and azathioprine therapy [see comments]. *Arth Rheum* 36: 1070–1079

107 Crilly A, McInness IB, McDonald AG, Watson J, Capell HA, Madhok R (1995) Interleukin 6 (IL-6) and soluble IL-2 receptor levels in patients with rheumatoid arthritis treated with low dose oral methotrexate. *J Rheumatol* 22: 224–226

108 Barrera P, Haagsma CJ, Boerbooms AMT, van Riel PLC, Borm GF, van de Putte LBA, van Der Meer JWM (1995) Effect of methotrexate alone or in combination with sulphasalazine on the production and circulating concentrations of cytokines and their antagonists. Longitudinal evaluation in patients with rheumatoid arthritis. *Br J Rheumatol* 34: 747–755

109 Barrera P, Boerbooms AM, Sauerwein RW, Demacker PN, van de Putte LB, van der Meer JW (1994) Interference of circulating azathioprine but not methotrexate or sulfasalazine with measurements of interleukin-6 bioactivity. *Lymphokine Cytokine Res* 13: 155–159

110 Seitz M, Loetscher P, Dewald B, Towbin H, Rordorf C, Gallati H, Baggiolini M, Gerber NJ (1995) Methotrexate action in rheumatoid arthritis: stimulation of cytokine inhibitor and inhibition of chemokine production by peripheral blood mononuclear cells. *Br J Rheumatol* 34: 602–609

111 Loetscher P, Dewald B, Baggiolini M, Seitz M (1994) Monocyte chemoattractant protein 1 and interleukin 8 production by rheumatoid synoviocytes. Effects of anti-rheumatic drugs. *Cytokine* 6: 162–170

112 Constantin A, Loubet-Lescoulie P, Lambert N, Yassine-Diab B, Abbal M, Mazieres B, de Preval C, Cantagrel A (1998) Antiinflammatory and immunoregulatory action of methotrexate in the treatment of rheumatoid arthritis: evidence of increased interleukin-4 and interleukin-10 gene expression demonstrated *in vitro* by competitive reverse transcriptase-polymerase chain reaction. *Arth Rheum* 41: 48–57

113 Merrill JT, Shen C, Schreibman D, Coffey D, Zakharenko O, Fisher R, Lahita RG, Salmon J, Cronstein BN (1997) Adenosine A_1 receptor promotion of multinucleated giant cell formation by human monocytes: a mechanism for methotrexate-induced nodulosis in rheumatoid arthritis. *Arth Rheum* 40: 1308–1315

114 Heenen M, Laporte M, Noel JC, de Graef C (1998) Methotrexate induces apoptotic cell death in human keratinocytes. *Arch Dermatol Res* 290: 240–245

115 Said S, Jeffes EW, Weinstein GD (1997) Methotrexate. *Clin Dermatol* 15: 781–797

Methotrexate in rheumatoid arthritis

Graciela S. Alarcón[1] and Sarah L. Morgan[2]

[1] *Multipurpose Arthritis and Musculoskeletal Diseases Center (MEB 615), The University of Alabama at Birmingham, Alabama, USA*
[2] *Nutrition Sciences Department (WEBB 212), The University of Alabama at Birmingham, Alabama, USA*

Introduction

Although a methotrexate (MTX) precursor, aminopterin, had been used for the treatment of arthritis (rheumatoid and psoriasis) in the 1950's [1, 2], the widespread utilization of MTX for the treatment of rheumatoid arthritis (RA) did not occur until the 1980's [3–5]. In this chapter, we will review the accepted issues regarding the use of this compound in RA as well as those issues which are less well accepted, but also of concern to the practicing rheumatologist. We will, for the most part, focus on adult patients with RA. The reader is referred to a number of publications dealing exclusively with children with juvenile (J) RA or JRA [6–12].

Efficacy

Anecdotal reports and small series reporting on the efficacy of MTX in RA were published in the 1980's [13–19] whereas randomized clinical trials (RCTs) were published in the mid 1980's [20–23]. A meta-analysis of these four pivotal trials published in 1987 clearly demonstrated the short term efficacy of the drug and contributed to its acceptance and approval as a treatment alternative for RA patients [24–26]. The long-term follow up of patients from these RCTs, as well as from other series, clearly demonstrated the sustained efficacy of this compound several years after its initiation [3, 27–36]. In fact, as compared to other disease-modifying anti-rheumatic drugs (DMARDs), our group as well as many others demonstrated that MTX had the highest retention rate at five years (around 50%) [36–44]. In contrast to other DMARDs, the beneficial effects of MTX are usually evident within weeks of its administration; thus corticosteroids as "bridge" therapy may be needed only for a short time [45]. Likewise, a severe flare occurs also within weeks of discontinuing it as demonstrated by Kremer et al. in a double-blind RCT [46]. Weinblatt et al. documented an increased frequency of HLA-DR2 among those patients who responded to MTX relative to normal controls in their initial RCT, but that observation was not validated in two other studies [22, 47, 48].

The ultimate efficacy of a compound in RA, however, should rest on its ability to influence not only those clinical features clearly related to persistent joint inflammation, but also to prevent the occurrence of joint destruction. A meta-analysis of the radiographic data on MTX-treated RA patients [49] failed to convincingly demonstrate that MTX could prevent the occurrence of joint destruction. The studies included in that meta-analysis, however, corresponded to the trials conducted in the early to mid 1980's in which patients with long-standing disease duration, who had previously failed one or more DMARDs, were enrolled [50–57]. Thus, it was felt that only by studying RA patients early in the course of their disease, and before joint destruction had occurred, that the ability of MTX to alter the destructive process could be definitively established. In fact, such data are now available. If MTX is used before joint erosions are present, patients are less likely to develop them than if they already have joint erosions prior to the initiation of MTX (30 and 70%, respectively in a study involving 24 patients) [58].

Toxicity

Towards the late 1980's our group recognized that toxicity, rather than lack of efficacy was the limiting factor in using MTX in RA patients [59, 60]. The most important predictors of MTX discontinuation were the occurrence of a toxic event and its severity [28]. Our group also recognized that the side effects produced by MTX were similar to complicated folate deficiency and could in fact be significantly ameliorated or prevented with the concomitant administration of folic acid. In fact, concurrent administration of other antifolates (such as trimethoprin-sulfamethoxazole) predisposes to MTX toxicity [35, 36, 38, 41, 61–63]. Doses of 5–27.5 mg of folic acid per week have been shown to lower toxicity without negating its efficacy [64, 65]. This practice has now been adopted by a sizable proportion of rheumatologists primarily in the Americas [66–69]. These folic acid supplementation studies also demonstrated that the efficacy of MTX is not altered by this therapeutic maneuver and thus the anti-rheumatic effects of this compound are not dependent upon the inhibition of the proximal enzymes in the folate pathway (such as dihydrofolate reductase) since folate levels increased durign folate supplementation. Low doses of folinic acid (a carbon substituted reduced folate) can also lower toxicity [70], however, larger doses negate efficacy which suggests the importance of folate pathways in the mechanism of efficacy [71]. We have hypothesized that inhibition of the distal enzymes in the folate pathway such as aminoimidazole carboxamide ribotide (AICAR) transformylase are necessary for efficacy [72]. The accumulation of AICAR, in turn, results in the accumulation of adenosine, a potent anti-inflammatory compound and possibly the basis for the anti-rheumatic effects of MTX are postulated by Cronstein et al. [73].

Other contributing factors to overall toxicity with MTX include decreased renal function and hypoalbuminemia [74]. Age and the use of nonsteroidal antiinflammatory drugs (NSAIDs) (aspirin included) are reported to be risk factors by some authors, but not by others [38, 75–83].

Standard methodology to report adverse events resulting from the administration of MTX was not available when our group conducted the folic acid supplementation RCTs. A toxicity score, which considered the severity, intensity, and duration of each toxic event was empirically derived and has proven useful in that context [64]; whether it may be applicable to clinical practice has not been determined.

It is not always possible to categorize MTX toxicities as being related to folate deficiency [59, 84, 85]. There are a few toxicities, however, which are clearly unrelated to folate deficiency and are more likely to be allergic reactions; that is the case for some skin rashes, post-dosing reactions, and pulmonary involvement [86]. Other side effects such as peripheral and visceral nodulosis are even harder to characterize. Thus, toxicities to MTX will be described *per* organ system with the exception of infection and malignant processes.

Hematopoietic system. Cytopenias of variable severity and involving one or all cell lines may occur in up to 25% of MTX-treated RA patients [63, 85, 87–97]. Although it has been postulated that cytopenias occurring with only a few doses of MTX are probably idiosyncratic [98], an underlying state of severe folate deficiency coupled with another contributing factor [concomitant administration of trimethoprin-sulfamethoxasole (another antifolate), or probenecid, hypoalbuminemia and/or renal insufficiency, for example], more than likely explains such occurrences [38, 62, 74, 87, 88, 90, 93, 97, 99–107]. Some published cases have been clearly related to dosing errors, a fact that should not be ignored (e.g. daily rather than weekly MTX ingestion) [108–111]. Severe cytopenias may require the administration of folinic acid (leucovorin rescue) and specific recombinant colony stimulating factors (much like those used in oncology) while mild cytopenias may respond simply to a dose reduction [67, 112] or the administration of folic acid [113].

Gastrointestinal (GI) tract. GI toxicities are rather common occurring in as many as 60% of patients [38, 59, 85, 89, 95, 114, 115]; they include stomatitis, anorexia, dyspepsia, nausea, vomiting and diarrhea and can be significantly curtailed either by reducing the dose of MTX or by administering folic acid. Upper and lower GI bleeding may result from severe mucosal involvement but in most cases other pharmacological compounds such as NSAIDs may be more directly implicated in inducing GI intolerance and bleeding. It has been stated that the parenteral administration of the compound may increase its GI tolerability, however that has not been rigorously examined.

Liver. MTX-induced liver toxicity was described in a quarter of patients with psoriasis treated with this compound [116]. Based on this experience, dermatologists established guidelines to monitor the administration of MTX [117]. We have not seen nearly as many adverse liver events as our dermatology colleagues, which more likely reflects the manner in which we administer MTX (weekly single dosing as opposed to every 12 h three times in psoriasis) and the adherence to a (very) limited (or nil) alcohol intake. While it is beyond doubt that MTX is hepatotoxic [118–135], probably as a result of its accumulation in the liver as polyglutamates [136], the important question is whether the histopathological abnormalities reported by light and electron microscopy correlate with liver disease of clinical importance or serious liver disease [128, 131, 134]. To this end, the work of Walker et al. on behalf of the American College of Rheumatology (ACR) deserves comment. This group not only established the probable frequency of clinically significant liver disease during low-dose MTX therapy for RA (one case per 1000 patients treated for five years) but also recognized the risk factors accounting for its occurrence (patient's age or age at MTX initiation and the duration of treatment or cumulative dose) [137]. Subsequently, Kremer et al. also on behalf of the ACR, drafted the currently available guidelines to monitor for hepatotoxicity in RA patients receiving MTX (*vide infra*) [138]. These authors emphasize the frequency with which liver function tests should be assayed, what to do if elevations of liver enzymes or a decrease in serum albumin levels occur, and when it is advisable (and cost-effective) to perform liver biopsies [134]. The risks (and cost) involved in performing liver biopsies were examined by Kremer et al. [138] and have been emphasized by other authors [139]. Subsequent work by other investigators have confirmed the value of the guidelines in terms of both risk factors and cost-effectiveness [133, 140–142]. It should be noted, however, that two possible additional risk factors have been identified; they are diabetes mellitus and heterozygous alpha 1-antitrypsin deficiency [133, 141, 142]. If liver biopsies are performed, the histo-pathological grading system as proposed by Roegnick et al. should be used [143]. Non-invasive radioisotope imaging studies are clearly inferior to liver biopsy to ascertain serious liver disease [144] and are currently not recommended. The role of ultrasound, single photon emission com-puterized tomography, magnetic resonance and computerized tomography in the detection of early liver involvement in these patients has not been established to date.

Respiratory system. Persistent cough without evidence of parenchymal lung involvement has been described in RA patients treated with MTX;

therefore, cough alone does not necessarily indicate an ensuing pneumonitis [145]. Pneumonitis, on the other hand, can be a very serious complication which should be promptly recognized and treated to prevent a fatal outcome [146]. It can occur even after very few doses of MTX intake [147, 148]. Criteria for the diagnosis of MTX-lung injury were first proposed by Searles and McKendry [149] and modified by the MTX-lung study group for their case-control study of risk factors for such an occurrence [150]. As shown in Table 1, these criteria are divided into major and minor categories. A definite diagnosis requires the presence of a major histopathological criterion or major radiological and microbiological criteria plus three minor criteria. A probable diagnosis of MTX-lung injury is made by the presence of major radiological and microbiological criteria and two minor criteria. All other cases are considered possible MTX-lung injury. The histopathological criterion requires not only an adequate tissue specimen, but the expertise of the pathologist in terms of features which may characterize RA and/or uncommon infections. Risk factors for lung involvement secondary to MTX administration identified by this group (and others with less sophisticated methods) using a multivariate domain logistic regression model included RA pleuropulmonary involvement, diabetes mellitus, hypoalbuminemia and age [62, 149–152].

Perhaps the most difficult clinical task is distinguishing MTX-lung from an opportunistic lung infection. Invasive studies, including bronchoalveolar lavage, closed lung biopsies and open lung biopsies for appropriate histopathological and microbiological studies (stains and cultures) may be required and they should be done without delay [62, 153–158]. In either situation (MTX-lung injury or infection), MTX is discontinued either temporarily (infection) or permanently (MTX-lung injury). If MTX-lung is

Table 1[a]. Adverse pulmonary events resulting from methotrexate therapy: revised diagnostic criteria[b]

Major criteria

1. Hypersensitivity pneumonitis by histopathology without evidence of pathogenic organisms
2. Radiological evidence of pulmonary interstitial or alveolar infiltrates
3. Blood cultures (if febrile) and initial sputum cultures (if sputum is produced) negative for pathogenic organisms

Minor criteria

1. Shortness of breath for < 8 weeks
2. Nonproductive cough
3. O_2 saturation $\leq 90\%$ at the time of initial evaluation on room air
4. $DL_{CO} \leq 70\%$ that predicted for age
5. Leukocyte count $\leq 15\,000$ cells/mm^3

[a] Reproduced with permission from [150].
[b] Adapted from Searles and McKendry [149]. DL_{CO} = diffusing capacity of the lung for carbon monoxide.

suspected, in addition to discontinuing MTX, supportive therapy, including high doses of corticosteroids, should be administered [147, 159–167]. Some patients succumb despite these and other measures such as ventilatory support. Patients who recover have been rechallenged with MTX successfully, however, half of the patients rechallenged may experience a fatal recurrence and thus MTX should not be restarted if a MTX-lung event has occurred [147].

Cardiovascular system. The administration of MTX, especially if folate supplementation is not provided, may result in hyperhomocysteinemia, a well recognized (independent) risk factor for atherosclerotic coronary artery and cerebrovascular diseases. Indeed, we showed increased levels of homocysteine in our early MTX-treated RA patients [168] as well as in our second folic acid supplementation study [132]. Patients on the placebo arm of the trial experienced impressive elevations of homocysteine levels, still another reason for folate supplementation. However we and others have not been able to document an increased prevalence of vascular (cerebral or cardiac) events in these patients [169].

Kidneys. Renal impairment is a significant contributing factor to the occurrence of toxicities in other organ systems, particularly the hematopoietic and GI systems [63, 81, 94, 106]. Whether MTX produces some degree of renal insufficiency has not been clearly established [170].

Central nervous system (CNS). A variety of CNS manifestations including headache, dizziness, vertigo, mood changes, seizures, ataxia and cognitive impairment have been infrequently described [59, 171, 172]. More ill-defined manifestations such as malaise and fatigue with or without arthralgias are not uncommon and could be central in origin [173]. A case of dementia occurring in temporal relationship with MTX administration (but which did not resolve after its discontinuation) has been reported [174].

Genitourinary (GU) tract. Erectile dysfunction, penile fibrosis and gynecomastia have been infrequently reported [175–177].

Reproductive system, pregnancy, contraception and fetal abnormalities. The current recommendation is to avoid conception (including impregnation) during MTX therapy and for three months after MTX has been discontinued. In our experience, unfortunately, many women become so incapacitated upon MTX discontinuation that, in fact, they do not become pregnant. Although an old report described five healthy neonates born to women who had received MTX during their pregnancy, five others were terminated by either spontaneous or therapeutic abortions [178]. More recently, a fetus with multiple abnormalities similar to the ones described as the "fetal aminopterin syndrome" has been reported [179]. In addition, folate deficiency has been recognized as playing a major role in the occurrence of neural tube defects and recommendations have been made to supplement flour with folic acid [180, 181] to prevent them. In short, MTX should be considered teratogenic and sexually active women (of childbearing age) and men (of any age) should be counseled so that a reliable method of contraception is used.

Musculoskeletal system. While an osteopathy has been documented in patients receiving MTX at chemotherapeutic doses [182], the role of MTX in the induction of osteoporosis (and osteoporotic fractures) at the doses used in RA remains debatable [183, 184]. While some case reports appear to confirm these side effects, larger series and even RCTs have failed to document these associations unless corticosteroids are also used [183, 185, 186]. A post-dosing reaction of variable severity and characterized by malaise and worsening arthralgias, similar to the one described in patients receiving gold salts, has been described [173]. The severe forms of this reaction are rather infrequent but may preclude the use of MTX in a small proportion of patients.

Integument. The use of MTX has been associated with the occurrence of alopecia, skin rashes and small vessel vasculitis [187–191]. Photosensitive reactions, porphyria cutanea tarda, toxicity from the concomitant use of topical 5-fluorouracil and nodulosis (*vide infra*) have also been described [192]. Onychomycosis and the occurrence of protracted skin cancers (in persons with a history of unprotected sun exposure) have been recognized by our group, although their frequency is unknown (unpublished observations).

Nodulosis. The appearance of crops of rather small (2–4 mm diameter) subcutaneous nodules (accelerated peripheral nodulosis) occurring in the palmar aspect of fingers and hands (or in the feet) is now a well recognized adverse event to the administration of MTX in both adults with RA and children with JRA [191, 193–196]. Their frequency is unknown and their exact pathogenesis is being elucidated [190, 197, 198]; unusual locations such as the penis have also been described [199]. Although these nodules are painless, they may significantly compromise fine motor function and add to the incapacitation already produced by the disease itself. Unfortunately, if removed surgically, these nodules tend to recur. Intervention with pharmacological compounds has been largely unsuccessful with the possible exception of sulphasalazine [200] and adenosine A1 receptor antagonists; the latter appear promising in *in vitro* studies [198].

Visceral nodulosis has been infrequently reported; locations include the myocardium, pericardium, pleura, lung and meningeal membranes [194, 197, 201–203]. The decision to discontinue MTX, if such a complication occurs, depends on whether or not organ system function is compromised.

MTX and malignancies. MTX has long been known to be a co-carcinogen, that is, it facilitates tumor growth and development in the presence of a defined carcinogenic substance (nicotine, for example). An increased occurrence of solid tumors and hematological malignancies in MTX-treated RA patients has not been consistently reported [204–206]. On the other hand, there are a substantial number of cases of rapidly growing lymphomas, some occurring in unusual locations (e.g. breast, palmar aspect of the hands, choroid and thigh), which may regress upon MTX discontinuation suggesting a clear cause and effect between MTX and their occurrence [89, 93, 207–225]. Most of the regressing lymphomas have been reported to be Epstein-Barr Virus (EBV)-related [212–214, 217]; two such cases have now been reported in children with JRA [226]. When these reports first appeared in the early 1990's, the (then) manufacturers of MTX recommended the issue be brought up for discussion before MTX was initiated. Despite these clinical data, the much larger body of epidemiological data suggests that the association between lymphomas and MTX is negligible [204, 206]. The clinician therefore has to carefully weigh whether or not to disclose this possible association to patients, taking into consideration the potential benefits for the joint disease.

MTX, infections and perioperative complications. There are data supporting the notion that RA patients receiving MTX experience a higher rate of common infections than those patients not treated with MTX [89, 227–230]. *In vitro* studies have not consistently supported the immunosuppressive action of MTX [231–236] in MTX-treated patients. However, there is an overwhelming body of evidence documenting the occurrence of opportunistic infections in these patients (Tab. 2) [154, 155, 237–255]. Thus, these patients should be treated properly and aggressively if infections ensue and the clinician should consider less common infections in these patients and proceed accordingly to diagnose them promptly and treat them properly.

Whether post-operative complications (infections and others such as delayed wound healing and wound dehiscence) occur with increased frequency in MTX-treated patients or not, is unresolved to date [256–264]. It is our practice, based on our own published data and experience, to withhold MTX for two weekly doses prior to and after elective orthopedic or abdominal surgery.

Table 2. Opportunistic pathogens and infectious processes reported in MTX-treated RA patients

Microorganism	Process/Organ involved	References
(1) Bacteria		
Pneumocistis Carinii	Pneumonia	[154, 243, 246–249, 251, 303, 304]
Listeria Monocytogenes	Bacteremia	[241]
	Meningitis	[59]
Atypical Mycobacteria	Lung	[246]
(2) Fungus		
Aspergillus	Lung	[244]
Histoplasmosis	Lung	[246]
Cyptococcocis	Pneumonia	[254]
Nocardia asteroides	Pneumonia	[305]
Candida albicans	Skin[a]	[109]
(3) Virus		
Herpes zoster	Disseminated	[242]
	Encephalomyelitis	[306]
Parvovirus	Red cell aplasia	[307]
Cytomegalovirus	Pneumonia	[155, 239]

[a] Patient had extensive skin necrosis secondary to acute MTX toxicity.

Administration

Route. The large majority of clinical, pharmacokinetic and pharmaco-dynamic studies have been done using oral MTX tablet administration [265, 266]. The use of the liquid form (for subcutaneous administration) orally [267] or the intramuscular route [268] have been advocated by some clinicians as less expensive and easier to administer forms of the compound; these advantages can not be disregarded. The use of MTX intra-articularly has been reported, but this route does not appear to be advantageous [269–271] and it is not used nowadays.

Dose. Since the initial MTX RCTs were published in the 1980's, rheumatologists have gained significant experience with dosing this compound. Most rheumatologists feel rather comfortable using doses much larger than the ones used in those initial studies (5–15 mg per week), especially when treating non-elderly adults. Starting doses of 10 mg per week, with a rapid escalation to a dose as high as 25 mg per week are not uncommon nowadays [89, 272, 273]. Some rheumatologists may push the dose even higher than 25 mg per week, if the drug is tolerated, and a full response has not been achieved. Whereas MTX was administered in the past in three divided doses given 12 hours apart, most MTX is now administered as a single dose [4]. Food probably does not affect the bioavailability of MTX although there are some data to the contrary [274, 275].

Baseline and subsequent ancillary evaluation. Prior to starting MTX, in addition to the baseline hematological and biochemical parameters, serologies for hepatitis B and C, and vitamin B_{12} levels are justified. Plasma and red blood cells (RBC) folate levels should be assayed if folate supplementation is not going to be started from the outset [138]. A chest radiograph should be strongly considered in the elderly, in men previously exposed to occupational or recreational toxins, and in patients with any suggestion of underlying bronchial or pleuro-parenchymal involvement [147]. Guidelines as to what tests to obtain (and how frequently), in order to anticipate untoward effects or detect them early have been established by the ACR [276] (Tab. 3).

Table 3. Recommended monitoring strategies for MTX administration*

Toxicities	Baseline	Follow-up	
		Symptoms/Examination	Ancillary
Myelosuppression	Complete blood cell (CBC) Plasma and RBC folate[a] Vitamin B_{12}[b]	Fever, Infections, Bruises	CBC and platelet count q 4–8 weeks
Hepatic fibrosis/ Cirrhosis	Hepatitis B and C serologies[c] AST/Aminoalamine transferase (ALT), Albumin Alkaline phosphatase		Aminospartate transferase (AST)/Albumin q 4–8 weeks
Renal impairment	Creatinine[d]		Creatinine q 4–8 weeks
Pneumonitis	Chest radiograph within one year	Shortness of breath (SOB), Persistent cough	
Lymphomas**		Lymph node enlargement	

 * Adapted from [276]; Less serious toxicities (e.g. stomatitis, alopecia, nausea, vomiting) are not included in this Table.
** Seems prudent to periodically monitor lymph node size.
[a] Only if no folate supplementation is to be given.
[b] Vitamin B_{12} deficiency may become overt with folate supplementation.
[c] Only on patients at risk.
[d] Renal impairment contributes to other toxic manifestations.

Folate supplementation. The work done by our group [64, 65, 70, 71, 277–280] and others [281], and elegantly examined by Ortiz et al. in a meta-analysis, clearly indicates that the concomitant administration of oxidized (folic acid) and reduced and carbon-substituted (folinic acid) forms of folate can decrease the toxicity to MTX [282]. Whereas folic acid can be administered at any time in relation to MTX and in any dose without concern at decreasing this drug's efficacy, that is not the case with folinic acid [64, 65, 277, 279, 283]. High doses of folinic acid and/or folinic acid administered close in time to MTX may decrease this drug's efficacy [71, 277]. In addition, at least in North America, folic acid is much cheaper than folinic acid and thus it is the preferred compound for supplementation. We use folic acid from the outset in all patients who are to receive MTX and reserve folinic acid for life-threatening side effects [68, 69, 284].

Early vs. late use of MTX. Our knowledge of the pathogenesis of RA and the limited "window of opportunity" for altering joint destruction in RA, is beyond the scope of this chapter [285, 286]. Most rheumatologists in the US, Canada and Latin America, are using MTX much earlier in the course of the disease than years ago [3, 37, 287–290].

Single vs. combined use of MTX. It is also beyond the scope of this chapter to discuss the use of MTX in conjunction with other DMARDs such as sulfasalazine (SASP) [291–294], gold salts, hydroxychloroquine (HCQ) [295], chloroquine [296], azathioprine [297, 298] or cyclosporine-A (Cs-A) [299–301]. Combination therapies which may pass the test of time may be those of MTX with HCQ, SASP and Cs-A. Furthermore, data on the combined use of MTX and the so-called biological compounds (anti-cytokine therapy) or newer DMARDs (leflunomide), are now being gathered. These combination therapies underscore the importance of understanding the mechanism of action of low dose MTX therapy.

Conclusions

Along with joint arthroplasties, MTX prescription has impacted dramatically on the lives of patients with RA. Only recently, new therapies have emerged which may offer beneficial effects in RA comparable to those of MTX (e.g. leflunomide) [302]. Until the efficacy-toxicity profile of leflunomide is recognized, or other therapeutic agents become available, and as we understand better the etiopathogenesis of this (often) devastating disease, it is very likely that MTX will continue to be used to treat these patients as it offers an adequate efficacy-toxicity profile.

References

1 Gubner R, August S, Ginsberg V (1951) Therapeutic suppression of tissue reactivity. II Effect of aminopterin in rheumatoid arthritis and psoriasis. *Am J Med Sci* 221:176–182.

2 Gubner R (1951) Therapeutic suppression of tissue reactivity. I. Comparison of the effects of cortisone and aminopterin. *Am J Med Sci* 221: 169–175

3 Rau R, Schleusser B, Herborn G, Karger T (1997) Longterm treatment of destructive rheumatoid arthritis with methotrexate. *J Rheumatol* 24: 1881–1889

4 Alarcón GS (1997) Methotrexate: Its use for the treatment of rheumatoid arthritis and other rheumatic disorders. In: WJ Koopman (ed): *Arthritis and Allied Conditions. A Textbook of Rheumatology*, Williams & Wilkins, Baltimore, 679–698

5 Bannwarth B, Vernhes J, Schaeverbeke T, Dehais J (1995) The facts about methotrexate in rheumatoid arthritis. *Rev Rheum* 62: 471–473

6 Rose CD, Singsen BH, Eichenfield AH, Goldsmith DP, Athreya BH (1990) Safety and efficacy of methotrexate therapy for juvenile rheumatoid arthritis. *J Pediatrics* 117: 653–659

7 White P, Ansell BM (1992) Methotrexate for juvenile rheumatoid arthritis. *N Engl J Med* 326: 1077–1078

8 Giannini EH, Brewer EJ, Kuzmina N, Shaikov A, Maximov A, Vorontsov I, Fink CW, Newman AJ, Cassidy JT, Zemel LS (1992) Methotrexate in resistant juvenile rheumatoid arthritis. Results of the U.S.A. – U.S.S.R. double-blind, placebo-controlled trial. *N Engl J Med* 326: 1043–1049

9 Graham LD, Myones BL, Rivas-Chacon RF, Pachman LM (1992) Morbidity associated with long-term methotrexate therapy in juvenile rheumatoid arthritis. *J Pediatrics* 120: 468–473

10 Wallace CA, Bleyer WA, Sherry DD, Salmonson KL, Wedgewood RJ (1989) Toxicity and serum levels of methotrexate in children with juvenile rheumatoid arthritis. *Arthritis Rheum* 32: 677–681

11 Singsen BH, Goldbach-Mansky R (1997) Methotrexate in the treatment of juvenile rheumatoid arthritis and other pediatric rheumatic and nonrheumatic disorders. *Rheum Dis Clin N Am* 23: 811–841

12 Harel L, Wagner-Weiner L, Poznanski AK, Spencer CH, Ekwo E, Magilavy DB (1993) Effects of methotrexate on radiologic progression in juvenile rheumatoid arthritis. *Arthritis Rheum* 36: 1370–1374

13 Hoffmeister RT (1983) Methotrexate therapy in rheumatoid arthritis: 15 years experience. *Am J Med* 75: 69–73

14 Willkens RF, Watson MA, Paxson CS (1980) Low dose pulse methotrexate therapy in rheumatoid arthritis. *J Rheumatol* 7: 501–505

15 Willkens RF (1983) Reappraisal of the use of methotrexate in rheumatic disease. *Am J Med* 75: 19–25

16 Michaels RM, Nashel DJ, Leonard A, Sliwinski AJ, Derbes SJ (1982) Weekly intravenous methotrexate in the treatment of rheumatoid arthritis. *Arthritis Rheum* 25: 339–341

17 Steinsson K, Weinstein A, Korn J, Abeles M (1982) Low dose methotrexate in rheumatoid arthritis. *J Rheumatol* 9: 860–866

18 Willkens RF, Watson MA (1982) Methotrexate: a perspective of its use in the treatment of rheumatic disease. *J Lab Clin Med* 100: 314–321

19 Wilke WS, Calabrese LH, Scherbel AL (1980) Methotrexate in the treatment of rheumatoid arthritis. Pilot study. *Cleve Clin Quart* 47: 305–309

20 Williams HJ, Willkens RF, Samuelson COJ, Alarcón GS, Guttadauria M, Yarboro C, Polisson RP, Weiner SR, Luggen ME, Billingsley LM, et al (1985) Comparison of low-dose oral pulse methotrexate and placebo in the treatment of rheumatoid arthritis. A controlled clinical trial. *Arthritis Rheum* 28: 721–730

21 Andersen PA, West SG, O'Dell JR, Via CS, Claypool RG, Kotzin BL (1985) Weekly pulse methotrexate in rheumatoid arthritis. Clinical and immunologic effects in a randomized, double-blind study. *Ann Intern Med* 103: 489–496

22 Weinblatt ME, Coblyn JS, Fox DA, Fraser PA, Holdsworth DE, Glass DN, Trentham DE (1985) Efficacy of low-dose methotrexate in rheumatoid arthritis. *N Engl J Med* 312: 818–822

23 Thompson RN, Watts C, Edelman J, Esdaile J, Russell AS (1984) A controlled two-centre trial of parenteral methotrexate therapy for refractory rheumatoid arthritis. *J Rheumatol* 11: 760–763

24 Tugwell P, Bennett K, Gent M (1987) Methotrexate in rheumatoid arthritis. Indications, contraindications, efficacy, and safety. *Ann Intern Med* 107: 358–366

25 Paulus HE (1986) FDA Arthritis Advisory Committee meeting: Methotrexate; guidelines for the clinical evaluation of antiinflammatory drugs; DMSO in scleroderma. *Arthritis Rheum* 29: 1289–1290

26 Health and Public Policy Committee HPPC, American College Physicians ACP (1987) Methotrexate in rheumatoid arthritis. *Ann Intern Med* 107: 418–419

27 Kremer JM (1997) Safety, efficacy, and mortality in a long-term cohort of patients with rheumatoid arthritis taking methotrexate: followup after a mean of 13.3 years. *Arthritis Rheum* 40: 984–985

28 Weinblatt ME, Kaplan H, Germain BF, Block S, Solomon SD, Merriman RC, Wolfe F, Wall B, Anderson L, Gall E, et al (1994) Methotrexate in rheumatoid arthritis: A five-year prospective multicenter study. *Arthritis Rheum* 37: 1492–1498

29 Kremer JM, Phelps CT (1992) Long-term prospective study of the use of methotrexate in the treatment of rheumatoid arthritis. Update after a mean of 90 months. *Arthritis Rheum* 35: 138–145

30 Weinblatt ME, Maier AL (1990) Longterm experience with low dose weekly methotrexate in rheumatoid arthritis. *J Rheumatol* 17: 33–38

31 Furst DE, Erikson N, Clute L, Koehnke R, Burmeister LF, Kohler JA (1990) Adverse experience with methotrexate during 176 weeks of a longterm prospective trial in patients with rheumatoid arthritis. *J Rheumatol* 17: 1628–1635

32 Weinblatt ME, Weissman BN, Holdsworth DE, Fraser PA, Maier AL, Falchuk KR, Coblyn JS (1992) Long-term prospective study of methotrexate in the treatment of rheumatoid arthritis. 84-month update. *Arthritis Rheum* 35: 129–137

33 Kremer JM, Lee JK (1992) A long-term prospective study of the use of methotrexate in rheumatoid arthritis. Update after a mean of fifty-three months. *Arthritis Rheum* 31: 577–584

34 Kremer JM, Lee JK (1986) The safety and efficacy of the use of methotrexate in long-term therapy for rheumatoid arthritis. *Arthritis Rheum* 29: 822–831

35 Salaffi F, Carotti M, Sartini A, Cervini C (1995) A prospective study of the long-term efficacy and toxicity of low-dose methotrexate in rheumatoid arthritis. *Clin Exp Rheumatol* 13: 23–28

36 Sany J, Anaya JM, Lussiez V, Couret M, Combe B, Daures JP (1991) Treatment of rheumatoid arthritis with methotrexate: a prospective open longterm study of 191 cases. *J Rheumatol*, 18: 1323–1327

37 Bologna C, Jorgensen C, Sany J (1997) Methotrexate as the initial second-line disease modifying agent in the treatment of rheumatoid arthritis patients. *Clin Exp Rheumatol* 15: 597–601

38 Tett SE, Triggs EJ (1996) Use of methotrexate in older patients. A risk-benefit assessment. *Drugs Aging* 9: 458–471

39 Wolfe F (1995) The epidemiology of drug treatment failure in rheumatoid arthritis. *Baillieres Clin Rheumatol* 9: 619–632

40 De La Mata J, Blanco FJ, Gomez-Reino JJ (1995) Survival analysis of disease modifying antirheumatic drugs in Spanish rheumatoid arthritis patients. *Ann Rheum Dis* 54: 881–885

41 Bannwarth B, Labat L, Moride Y, Schaeverbeke T (1994) Methotrexate in rheumatoid arthritis. An update. *Drugs* 47: 25–50

42 Pincus T, Callahan LF (1993) Variability in individual responses of 532 patients with rheumatoid arthritis to first-line and second-line drugs. *Agents Actions* (Supplement) 40: 67–75

43 Buchbinder R, Hall S, Sambrook PN, Champion GD, Harkness A, Lewis D, Littlejohn GO, Miller MH, Ryan PFJ (1993) Methotrexate therapy in rheumatoid arthritis: A life table review of 587 patients treated in community practice. *J Rheumatol* 20: 639–644

44 Wolfe F, Hawley DJ, Cathey MA (1990) Termination of slow acting antirheumatic therapy in rheumatoid arthritis. A 14-year prospective evaluation of 1017 consecutive starts. *J Rheumatol* 17: 994–1002

45 Van der Veen MJ, Bijlsma JW (1993) The effect of methylprednisolone pulse therapy on methotrexate treatment of rheumatoid arthritis. *Clin Rheumatol* 12: 500–505

46 Kremer JM, Rynes RI, Bartholomew LE (1987) Severe flare of rheumatoid arthritis after discontinuation of long-term methotrexate therapy. Double-blind study. *Am J Med* 82: 781–786

47 Alarcón GS, Guyton JM, Acton RT, Barger BO, Koopman WJ (1986) DR2 positivity and response to methotrexate in rheumatoid arthritis. *Arthritis Rheum* 29: 151

48 Alarcón GS, Billingsley LM, Clegg DO, Hardin JG, Klippel J, Luggen ME, Polisson RP, Singer JZ, Szydlo L, Willkens RF, et al (1987) Lack of association between HLA-DR2 and clinical response to methotrexate in patients with rheumatoid arthritis. *Arthritis Rheum* 30: 218–220

49 Alarcón GS, López-Méndez A, Walter J, Boerbooms AMT, Russell AS, Furst DE, Rau R, Drosos AA, Bartolucci AA (1992) Radiographic evidence of disease progression in methotrexate treated and nonmethotrexate disease modifying antirheumatic drug treated rheumatoid arthritis patients: A meta-analysis. *J Rheumatol* 19: 1868–1873

50 López-Méndez A, Daniel WW, Reading JC, Ward JR, Alarcón GS (1993) Radiographic assessment of disease progression in rheumatoid arthritis patients enrolled in the co-operative systemic studies of the rheumatic diseases program randomized clinical trial of methotrexate, auranofin, or a combination of the two. *Arthritis Rheum* 36: 1364–1369

51 Weinblatt ME, Polisson R, Blotner SD, Sosman JL, Aliabadi P, Baker N, Weissman BN (1993) The effects of drug therapy on radiographic progression of rheumatoid arthritis. Results of a 36-week randomized trial comparing methotrexate and auranofin. *Arthritis Rheum* 36: 613–619

52 Jeurissen MEC, Boerbooms MT, van de Putte LBA, Doesburg WH, Lemmens AM (1991) Influence of methotrexate and azathioprine on radiologic progression in rheumatoid arthritis. A randomized, double-blind study. *Ann Intern Med* 114: 999–1004

53 Sany J, Kaliski S, Couret M, Cuchacovich M, Daures J (1990) Radiologic progression during intramuscular methotrexate treatment of rheumatoid arthritis. *J Rheumatol* 17: 1636–1641

54 Drosos AA, Karantanas AH, Psychos D, Tsampoulas C, Moutsopoulos HM (1990) Can treatment with methotrexate influence the radiological progression of rheumatoid arthritis? *Clin Rheumatol* 9: 342–345

55 Reykdal S, Steinsson K, Sigurjonsson K, Brekkan A (1989) Methotrexate treatment of rheumatoid arthritis: Effects on radiological progression. *Scand J Rheumatol*, 18:221-226

56 Hanrahan PS, Scrivens GA, Russell AS (1989) Prospective long-term follow-up of methotrexate therapy in rheumatoid arthritis: toxicity, efficacy and radiological progression. *Br J Rheumatol* 28: 147–153

57 Nordstrom DM, West SG, Andersen PA, Sharp JT (1987) Pulse methotrexate therapy in rheumatoid arthritis. A controlled prospective roentgenographic study. *Ann Intern Med* 107: 797–801

58 Rich E, Moreland LW, Alarcón GS (1999) Paucity of radiographic progression in rheumatoid arthritis treated with methotrexate as the first disease-modifying anti-rheumatid drug. *J Rheumatol* 26: 259–261

59 Gispen JG, Alarcón GS, Johnson JJ, Acton RT, Barger BO, Koopman WJ (1987) Toxicity to methotrexate in rheumatoid arthritis. *J Rheumatol* 14: 74–79

60 Alarcón GS, Tracy IC, Blackburn WDJ (1989) Methotrexate in rheumatoid arthritis. Toxic effects as the major factor in limiting long-term treatment. *Arthritis Rheum* 32: 671–676

61 Groenendal H, Rampen FH (1990) Methotrexate and trimethoprim-sulphamethoxazole – a potentially hazardous combination. *Clin Exp Dermatol* 15: 358–360

62 Berthelot JM, Glemarec J, Chiffoleau A, Maugars Y, Prost A (1997) Treatment with low dose methotrexate in rheumatoid arthritis: risk factors for severe complications. [Traitements a faibles doses par le methotrexate dans la polyarthrite rheumatoide: facteurs de risque des complications graves]. *Therapie* 52: 111–118

63 Bruyn GA, Velthuysen E, Joosten P, Houtman PM (1995) Pancytopenia related eosino-philia in rheumatoid arthritis: a specific methotrexate phenomenon? *J Rheumatol* 22: 1373–1376

64 Morgan SL, Baggott JE, Vaughn WH, Young PK, Austin JV, Krumdieck CL, Alarcón GS, Koopman WJ (1990) The effect of folic acid supplementation on the toxicity of low-dose methotrexate in patients with rheumatoid arthritis. *Arthritis Rheum* 33: 9–18

65 Morgan SL, Baggott JE, Vaughn WH, Austin JS, Veitch TA, Lee JY, Koopman WJ, Krumdieck CL, Alarcón GS (1994) Supplementation with folic acid during methotrexate therapy for rheumatoid arthritis. A double-blind, placebo-controlled trial. *Ann Intern Med* 121: 833–841

66 Gulko PS, Tracy IC, Baum SK, Hsu W, Morgan SL, Alarcón GS (1994) Practice patterns in the use of supplemental folic acid in rheumatoid arthritis patients treated with methotrexate. *Rev Brasil Rheumatol* 34: 235–238

67 Jobanputra P, Hunter M, Clark D, Lambert CM, Hurst NP (1995) An audit of methotrexate and folic acid for rheumatoid arthritis. Experience from a teaching centre. *Br J Rheumatol* 34: 971–975

68 Morgan SL, Baggott JE, Alarcón GS (1997) Methotrexate in rheumatoid arthritis. Folate supplementation should always be given. *BioDrugs* 8: 164–175

69 Morgan SL, Alarcón GS, Krumdieck CL (1993) Folic acid supplementation during methotrexate therapy: It makes sense. *J Rheumatol* 20: 929–930

70 Buckley LM, Vacek PM, Cooper SM (1990) Administration of folinic acid after low dose methotrexate in patients with rheumatoid arthritis. *J Rheumatol* 17: 1158–1161

71 Joyce DA, Will RK, Hoffman DM, Laing B, Blackbourn SJ (1991) Exacerbation of rheumatoid arthritis in patients treated with methotrexate after administration of folinic acid. *Ann Rheum Dis* 50: 913–914

72 Baggott JE, Morgan SL, Ha T, Alarcón GS, Koopman WJ, Krumdieck CL (1993) Antifolates in rheumatoid arthritis: a hypothetical mechanism of action. *Clin Exp Rheumatol* 11: S101–S105

73 Cronstein BN (1997) The mechanism of action of methotrexate. *Rheum Dis Clin N Am* 23: 739–755

74 Doolittle GC, Simpson KM, Lindsley HB (1989) Methotrexate-associated, early-onset pancytopenia in rheumatoid arthritis. *Arch Intern Med* 149: 1430–1431

75 Bressolle F, Bologna C, Kinowski JM, Arcos B, Sany J, Combe B (1997) Total and free methotrexate pharmacokinetics in elderly patients with rheumatoid arthritis. A comparison with young patients. *J Rheumatol* 24: 1903–1909

76 Biasi D, Carletto A, Caramaschi P, Bambara LM (1996) Efficacy and safety of low dose methotrexate in elderly onset rheumatoid arthritis. *J Rheumatol* 23: 407–408

77 Wolfe F, Cathey MA (1991) The effect of age on methotrexate efficacy and toxicity. *J Rheumatol* 18: 973–979

78 Fries JF, Singh G, Lenert L, Furst DE (1990) Aspirin, hydroxychloroquine, and hepatic enzyme abnormalities with methotrexate in rheumatoid arthritis. *Arthritis Rheum* 33: 1611–1619

79 Rooney TW, Furst DE, Koehnke R, Burmeister L (1993) Aspirin is not associated with more toxicity than other nonsteroidal antiinflammatory drugs in patients with rheumatoid arthritis treated with methotrexate. *J Rheumatol* 20: 1297–1302

80 Stewart CF, Fleming RA, Germain BF, Seleznick MJ, Evans WE (1991) Aspirin alters methotrexate disposition in rheumatoid arthritis patients. *Arthritis Rheum* 34: 1514–1520

81 Anonymous (1995) The effect of age and renal function on the efficacy and toxicity of methotrexate in rheumatoid arthritis. Rheumatoid Arthritis Clinical Trial Archive Group. *J Rheumatol* 22: 218–223

82 Wallace CA, Smith AL, Sherry DD (1993) Pilot investigation of naproxen/methotrexate interaction in patients with juvenile rheumatoid arthritis. *J Rheumatol* 20: 1764–1768

83 Furst DE (1995) Practical clinical pharmacology and drug interactions of low-dose methotrexate therapy in rheumatoid arthritis. *Br J Rheumatol* 34: 20–25

84 McKendry RJR (1997) The remarkable spectrum of methotrexate toxicities. *Rheum Dis Clin N Am* 23: 939–955

85 McKendry RJR, Dale P (1993) Adverse effects of low dose methotrexate therapy in rheumatoid arthritis. *J Rheumatol* 20: 1850–1856

86 Sandoval DM, Alarcón GS, Morgan SL (1995) Adverse events in methotrexate-treated rheumatoid arthritis patients. *Br J Rheumatol* 34: 49–56

87 Laroche F, Perrot S, Menkes CJ (1996) Pancytopenia in rheumatoid arthritis treated with methotrexate. [Pancytopenies au cours de la polyarthrite rhumatoide traitee par methotrexate]. *Presse Medicale* 25: 1144–1146

88 Franck H, Rau R, Herborn G (1996) Thrombocytopenia in patients with rheumatoid arthritis on long-term treatment with low dose methotrexate. *Clin Rheumatol* 15: 266–270

 89 Schnabel A, Herlyn K, Burchardi C, Reinhold-Keller E, Gross WL (1996) Long-term tol-
    erability of methotrexate at doses exceeding 15 mg per week in rheumatoid arthritis. *Rheu-
    matol Internatl* 15: 195–200
 90 Gutierrez-Ureña S, Molina JF, García CO, Cuéllar ML, Espinoza LR (1996) Pancytopenia
    secondary to methotrexate therapy in rheumatoid arthritis. *Arthritis Rheum* 39: 272–276
 91 Myllykangas-Luosujärvi R, Aho K, Isomäki H (1995) Death attributed to antirheumatic
    medication in a nationwide series of 1666 patients with rheumatoid arthritis who have
    died. *J Rheumatol* 22: 2214–2217
 92 Berthelot J, Maugars Y, Hamidou M, Chiffoleau A, Barrier J, Gorolleau J, Prost A (1995)
    Pancytopenia and severe cytopenia induced by low-dose methotrexate. Eight case-reports
    and a review of one hundred cases from the literature (with twenty-four deaths). *Rev
    Rheum* (English Edition) 62: 477–486
 93 Trenkwalder P, Eisenlohr H, Prechtel K, Lydtin H (1992) Three cases of malignant
    neoplasm, pneumonitis, and pancytopenia during treatment with low-dose methotrexate.
    Clin Investig 70: 951–955
 94 Mayall B, Poggi G, Parkin JD (1991) Neutropenia due to low-dose methotrexate therapy
    for psoriasis and rheumatoid arthritis may be fatal. *Med J Australia* 155: 480–484
 95 Drosos AA, Psychos D, Andonopoulos AP, Stefanaki-Nikou S, Tsianos EB (1990)
    Methotrexate therapy in rheumatoid arthritis. A two year prospective follow-up. *Clin
    Rheumatol* 9: 333–341
 96 Szanto E (1989) Low-dose methotrexate treatment of rheumatoid arthritis; long-term
    observation of efficacy and safety. *Clin Rheumatol* 8: 323–330
 97 Mackinnon SK, Starkebaum G, Willkens RF (1985) Pancytopenia associated with low
    dose pulse methotrexate in the treatment of rheumatoid arthritis. *Sem Arthritis Rheum* 15:
    119–126
 98 Tanaka Y, Shiozawa K, Nishibayashi Y, Imura S (1992) Methotrexate induced early onset
    pancytopenia in rheumatoid arthritis: Drug allergy? Idiosyncrasy? *J Rheumatol* 19:
    1320–1321
 99 Maricic M, Davis M, Gall EP (1986) Megaloblastic pancytopenia in a patient receiving
    concurrent methotrexate and trimethoprim-sulfamethoxazole treatment. *Arthritis Rheum*
    29: 133–135
100 Al-Awadhi A, Dale P, McKendry RJR (1993) Pancytopenia associated with low dose
    methotrexate therapy. *J Rheumatol* 20: 1121–1124
101 Casserly CM, Stange KC, Chren MM (1993) Severe megaloblastic anemia in a patient
    receiving low-dose methotrexate for psoriasis. *J Am Acad Dermatol* 29: 477–480
102 Thomas MH, Gutterman LA (1986) Methotrexate toxicity in a patient receiving trimetho-
    prim-sulfamethoxazole. *J Rheumatol* 13: 440–441
103 Basin KS, Escalante A, Beardmore TD (1991) Severe pancytopenia in a patient taking low
    dose methotrexate and probenecid. *J Rheumatol* 18: 608–610
104 Noskov SM (1990) Megaloblastic pancytopenia in a female patient with rheumatoid
    arthritis given methotrexate and amidopyrine simultaneously. [Megaloblasticheskaia pant-
    sitopeniia u bol'noi revmatoidnym artritom pri odnovremennom primeneniem meto-
    treksata i amidopirina]. *Terapevticheskii Arkhiv*, 62: 122–123
105 Weinblatt ME, Fraser P (1989) Elevated mean corpuscular volume as a predictor of
    hematologic toxicity due to methotrexate therapy. *Arthritis Rheum* 32: 1592–1596
106 Kevat SG, Hill WR, McCarthy PJ, Ahern MJ (1988) Pancytopenia induced by low-dose
    methotrexate for rheumatoid arthritis. *Aust NZ J Med* 18: 697–700
107 Thevenet JP, Ristori JM, Cure H, Mizony MH, Bussiere JL (1987) Pancytopenia during
    treatment of rheumatoid arthritis with methotrexate after administration of trimethoprim-
    sulfamethoxazole. [Pancytopenie au cours du traitement d'une polyarthrite rheumatoide
    par methotrexate apres administration de trimethoprime-sulfamethoxazole]. *Presse Medi-
    cale* 16: 1487
108 Maignen F, Guillot B, Pierron E, Julian S, Castot A (1996) Acute methotrexate poisoning:
    apropos of 16 cases reported to the Paris Poison Control Center and review of the
    literature. [L'intoxication aigue au methotrexate: a propos de 16 cas rapportes au Centre
    Anti-Poisons de Paris et revue de la litterature]. *Therapie* 51: 527–531
109 Porawska W (1995) Overdose of methotrexate with a fatal outcome in a patient with
    rheumatoid arthritis. [Przedawkowanie metotreksatu przyczyna zgonu chorej na
    reumatoidalne zapalenie stawow]. *Polskie Archi Med Wewnet* 93: 346–350

110 Brown MA, Corrigan AB (1991) Pancytopenia after accidental overdose of methotrexate. A complication of low-dose therapy for rheumatoid arthritis. *Med J Aust* 155: 493–494

111 Lomaestro BM, Lesar TS, Hager TP (1992) Errors in prescribing methotrexate. *J Am Med Asso* 268: 2031–2032

112 Stenger AAME, Houtman PM, Bruyn GAW (1992) Does folate supplementation make sense in patients with rheumatoid arthritis treated with methotrexate? *Ann Rheum Dis* 51: 1019–1020

113 Bolla G, Disdier P, Harle JR, Verrot D, Weiller PJ (1993) Concurrent acute megaloblastic anaemia and pneumonitis: a severe side-effect of low-dose methotrexate therapy during rheumatoid arthritis. *Clin Rheumatol* 12: 535–537

114 Ince A, Yazici Y, Hamuryudan V, Yazici H (1996) The frequency and clinical characteristics of methotrexate (MTX) oral toxicity in rheumatoid arthritis (RA) a masked and controlled study. *Clin Rheumatol* 15: 491–494

115 Klippel JH, Strober S, Wofsy D (1989) New therapies for the rheumatic diseases. *Bulletin Rheum Dis* 38: 1–7

116 Dahl MGC, Gregory MM, Scheuer PJ (1972) Methotrexate hepatotoxicity in psoriasis-comparison of different dose regimens. *Br Med J* 1: 654–656

117 Robinson JK, Baughman RD, Auerbach R, Cimis RJ (1980) Methotrexate hepatotoxicity in psoriasis. Consideration of liver biopsies at regular intervals. *Arch Dermatol* 116: 413–415

118 ter Borg EJ, Seldenrijk CA, Timmer R (1996) Liver cirrhosis due to methotrexate in a patient with rheumatoid arthritis. *Netherlands J Med* 49: 244–246

119 Bjorkman DJ, Boschert M, Tolman KG, Clegg DO, Ward JR (1993) The effect of long-term methotrexate therapy on hepatic fibrosis in rheumatoid arthritis. *Arthritis Rheum* 36: 1691–1696

120 Minocha A, Dean HA, Pittsley RA (1993) Liver cirrhosis in rheumatoid arthritis patients treated with long-term methotrexate. *Vet Human Toxicol* 35: 45–48

121 Phillips CA, Cera PJ, Mangan TF, Newman ED (1992) Clinical liver disease in patients with rheumatoid arthritis taking methotrexate. *J Rheumatol* 19: 229–233

122 Ahern MJ, Kevat S, Hill W, Hayball PJ, Harley H, Hall P (1991) Hepatic methotrexate content and progression of hepatic fibrosis: preliminary findings. *Ann Intern Med* 50: 477–480

123 White-O'keefe QE, Fye KH, Sack KD (1991) Methotrexate and histologic abnormalities: A meta-analysis. *Am J Med* 70: 711–716

124 Kujala GA, Shamma'A JM, Chang WL, Brick JE (1990) Hepatitis with bridging fibrosis and reversible hepatic insufficiency in a woman with rheumatoid arthritis taking methotrexate. *Arthritis Rheum* 33: 1037–1041

125 Clegg DO, Furst DE, Tolman KG, Pogue R (1989) Acute, reversible hepatic failure associated with methotrexate treatment of rheumatoid arthritis. *J Rheumatol* 16: 1123–1126

126 Bjorkman DJ, Hammond EH, Lee RG, Clegg DO, Tolman KG (1988) Hepatic ultrastructure after methotrexate therapy for rheumatoid arthritis. *Arthritis Rheum* 31: 1465–1472

127 Aponte J, Petrelli M (1988) Histopathologic findings in the liver of rheumatoid arthritis patients treated with long-term bolus methotrexate. *Arthritis Rheum* 31: 1457–1464

128 Kremer JM, Lee RG, Tolman KG (1989) Liver histology in rheumatoid arthritis patients receiving long-term methotrexate therapy. A prospective study with baseline and sequential biopsy samples. *Arthritis Rheum* 32: 121–127

129 Shergy WJ, Polisson RP, Caldwell DS, Rice JR, Pisetsky DS, Allen NB (1988) Methotrexate-associated hepatotoxicity: retrospective analysis of 210 patients with rheumatoid arthritis. *Am J Med* 85: 711–774

130 Leonard PA, Clegg DO, Carson CC, Cannon GW, Egger MJ, Ward JR (1987) Low dose pulse methotrexate in rheumatoid arthritis: an 8-year experience with hepatotoxicity. *Clin Rheumatol* 6: 575–582

131 Kremer JM, Kaye GI, Kaye NW, Kamal IG, Axiotis CA (1995) Light and electron microscopic analysis of sequential liver biopsy samples for rheumatoid arthritis patients receiving long-term methotrexate therapy: Follow-up over long treatment intervals and correlation with clinical and laboratory variables. *Arthritis Rheum* 38: 1194–1203

132 Morgan SL, Baggott JE, Lee JY, Alarcón GS (1998) Folic acid supplementation prevents deficient blood folate levels and hyperhomocysteinemia during longterm, low dose methotrexate therapy for rheumatoid arthritis: Implications for cardiovascular disease prevention. *J Rheumatol* 25: 441–446

133 West SG (1997) Methotrexate hepatotoxicity. *Rheum Dis Clin N Am* 23: 883–915

134 Kremer JM, Furst DE, Weinblatt ME, Blotner SD (1996) Significant changes in serum AST across hepatic histological biopsy grades: Prospective analysis of 3 cohorts receiving methotrexate therapy for rheumatoid arthritis. *J Rheumatol* 23: 459–460

135 Bridges SLJ, Alarcón GS, Koopman WJ (1989) Methotrexate-induced liver abnormalities in rheumatoid arthritis. *J Rheumatol* 16: 1180–1183

136 Kremer JM, Galivan J, Streckfuss A, Kamen B (1986) Methotrexate metabolism analysis in blood and liver of rheumatoid arthritis patients. Association with hepatic folate deficiency and formation of polyglutamates. *Arthritis Rheum* 29: 832–835

137 Walker AM, Funch D, Dreyer NA, Tolman KG, Kremer JM, Alarcón GS, Lee RG, Weinblatt ME (1993) Determinants of serious liver disease among patients receiving low-dose methotrexate for rheumatoid arthritis. *Arthritis Rheum* 36: 329–335

138 Kremer JM, Alarcón GS, Lightfoot RW Jr, Willkens RF, Furst DE, Williams HJ (1994) Methotrexate for rheumatoid arthritis. Suggested guidelines for monitoring liver toxicity. *Arthritis Rheum* 37: 316–328

139 Cash JM, Swain M, Di Bisceglie M, Wilder RL, Crofford LJ (1992) Massive intrahepatic hemorrhage following routine liver biopsy in a patient with rheumatoid arthritis treated with methotrexate. *J Rheumatol* 19: 1466–1468

140 Bergquist SR, Felson DT, Prashker MJ, Freedberg KA (1995) The cost-effectiveness of liver biopsy in rheumatoid arthritis patients treated with methotrexate. *Arthritis Rheum* 38: 326–333

141 Erickson AR, Reddy V, Vogelgesang SA, West SG (1995) Usefulness of the American College of Rheumatology recommendations for liver biopsy in methotrexate-treated rheumatoid arthritis patients. *Arthritis Rheum* 38: 1115–1119

142 Hilsden RJ, Urbanski SJ, Swain MG (1995) End-stage liver disease developing with the use of methotrexate in heterozygous α1-antitrypsin deficiency. *Arthritis Rheum* 38: 1014–1018

143 Roenigk HH Jr, Maibach HI, Auerbach R, Weinstein GD (1982) Methotrexate guidelines – revised. *J Am Acad Dermatol* 6: 145–155

144 Arias JM, Morton KA, Albro JE, Patch GG, Valdivia S, Greenberg HE, Christian PE, Datz FL (1993) Comparison of methods for identifying early methotrexate-induced hepatotoxicity in patients with rheumatoid arthritis. *J Nucl Med* 34: 1905–1909

145 Schnabel A, Dalhoff K, Bauerfeind S, Barth J, Gross WL (1996) Sustained cough in methotrexate therapy for rheumatoid arthritis. *Clin Rheumatol* 15: 277–282

146 Hilliquin P, Renoux M, Perrot S, Puechal X, Menkes CJ (1996) Occurrence of pulmonary complications during methotrexte therapy in rheumatoid arthritis. *Br J Rheumatol* 35: 441–445

147 Kremer JM, Alarcón GS, Kaymakcian M, Macaluso M, Weinblatt ME, Cannon GW, Palmer WR, Sundy JS, Golden HF, Alexander RW, et al (1997) Clinical, laboratory radiographic and histopathological features of methotrexate-associated lung injury in patients with rheumatoid arthritis: A multicenter study with literature review. *Arthritis Rheum* 40: 1829–1837

148 Van der Veen MJ, Dekker JJ, Dinant HJ, van Soesbegen RM, Bijlsma JW (1995) Fatal pulmonary fibrosis complicating low dose methotrexate therapy for rheumatoid arthritis. *J Rheumatol* 22: 1766–1768

149 Searles G, McKendry RJR (1987) Methotrexate pneumonitis in rheumatoid arthritis: Potential risk factors. Four case reports and a review of the literature. *J Rheumatol* 14: 1164–1171

150 Alarcón GS, Kremer JM, Macaluso M, Weinblatt ME, Cannon GW, Palmer WR, St Clair EW, Sundy JS, Alexander RW, et al (1997) Risk factors for methotrexate-induced lung injury in patients with rheumatoid arthritis. A multicenter, case-control study. Methotrexate-Lung Study Group. *Ann Intern Med* 127: 356–364

151 Golden MR, Katz RS, Balk RA, Golden HE (1995) The relationship of preexisting lung disease to the development of methotrexate pneumonitis in patients with rheumatoid arthritis. *J Rheumatol* 22: 1043–1047

152 Carroll GJ, Thomas R, Phatouros CC, Atchison MH, Leslie AL, Cook NJ, D'Souza I (1994) Incidence, prevalence and possible risk factors for pneumonitis in patients with rheumatoid arthritis receiving methotrexate. *J Rheumatol* 21: 51–54

153 Schnabel A, Richter C, Bauerfeind S, Gross WL (1997) Bronchoalvelolar lavage cell profile in methotrexate induced pneumonitis. *Thorax* 52: 377–379

154 Roux N, Flipo RM, Cortet B, Lafitte JJ, Tonnel AB, Duquesnoy B, Delcambre B (1996) Pneumocystis carinii pneumonia in rheumatoid arthritis patients treated with methotrexate. A report of two cases. *Revue Du Rhum*, 63: 453–456

155 Aglas R, Rainer F, Hermann J, Gretler J, Huttl E, Domej W, Krejs GJ (1995) Interstitial pneumonia due to cytomegalovirus following low-dose methotrexate treatment for rheumatoid arthritis. *Arthritis Rheum*, 38: 291–292

156 St.Clair EW, Rice JR, Snyderman R (1985) Pneumonitis complicating low-dose methotrexate therapy in rheumatoid arthritis. *Arch Intern Med* 145: 2035–2038

157 Law KF, Aranda CP, Smith RL, Berkwoitz KA, Ittman MM, Lewis ML (1993) Pulmonary cryptococcosis mimicking methotrexate pneumonitis. *J Rheumatol* 20: 872–873

158 White DA, Rankin JA, Stover DE, Gellene RA, Gupta S (1989) Methotrexate pneumonitis. Bronchoalveolar lavage findings suggest an immunologic disorder. *Am Rev Resp Dis* 139: 18–21

159 Massin F, Coudert B, Marot JP, Foucher P, Camus P, Jeannin L (1990) Pneumopathy caused by methotrexate. [La pneumopathie du methotrexate]. *Rev Maladies Resp* 7: 5–15

160 Hand SH, Smith JK, Chaudhary BA (1989) Methotrexate pneumonitis: a case report and summary of the literature. *J Med Assoc GA* 78: 625–628

161 Green L, Schattner A, Berkenstadt H (1988) Severe reversible interstitial pneumonitis induced by low dose methotrexate: report of a case and review of the literature. *J Rheumatol*, 15:110-112

162 Cottin V, Tebib J, Massonnet B, Souquet PJ, Bernard JP (1997) Respiratory function surveillance during prolonged treatment with low-dose methotrexate. [La surveillance fonctionnelle respiratoire au cours d'un traitement prolonge par le methotrexate a faible dose]. *Presse Medicale* 26: 404–406

163 Anaya J, Diethelm L, Ortiz LA, Gutierrez M, Citera G, Welsh RA, Espinoza LR (1995) Pulmonary involvement in rheumatoid arthritis. *Sem Arthritis Rheum* 24: 242–254

164 Carson CW, Cannon GW, Egger MJ, Ward JR, Clegg DO (1987) Pulmonary disease during the treatment of rheumatoid arthritis with low dose pulse methotrexate. *Sem Arthritis Rheum* 16: 186–195

165 Tugwell P, Bombardier C, Buchanan WW, Goldsmith C, Grace E, Bennett KJ, Williams HJ, Egger M, Alarcón GS, Guttadauria M, et al (1990) Methotrexate in rheumatoid arthrits. Impact on quality of life assessed by traditional standard-item and individualized patient preference health status questionnaires. *Arch Intern Med* 150: 59–62

166 Elasser S, Dalquen P, Soler M, Perrachoud AP (1989) Methotrexate-induced pneumonitis: appearance four weeks after discontinuation of treatment. *Am Rev Resp Dis* 140: 1089–1092

167 Quadri F, Marone C (1989) Schwere akute Pneumopathie nach low-dose-methotrexate-therapie bei chronischer Polyarthritis [Acute peumonitis after low dose methotrexate therapy for chronic polyarthritis]. *Schweiz Med Wschr* 119: 1434–1436

168 Morgan SL, Baggott JE, Refsum H, Ueland PM (1991) Homocysteine levels in patients with rheumatoid arthritis treated with low-dose methotrexate. *Clin Pharmacol Therapeu* 50: 547–556

169 Alarcón GS, Tracy IC, Strand GM, Singh K, Macaluso M (1995) Survival and drug discontinuation analyses in a large cohort of methotrexate-treated rheumatoid arthritis patients. *Ann Rheum Dis* 54: 708–712

170 Seideman P, Muller-Suur R, Ekman E (1998) Renal effects of low dose methotrexate in rheumatoid arthritis. *J Rheumatol* 20: 1126–1128

171 Thomas E, Leroux JL, Hellier JP, Blotman F (1993) Seizure and methotrexate therapy in rheumatoid arthritis. *J Rheumatol* 20: 1632

172 Wernick R, Smith DL (1989) Central nervous system toxicity associated with weekly low-dose methotrexate treatment. *Arthritis Rheum* 32: 770–775

173 Halla JT, Hardin JG (1994) Underreccognized postdosing reactions to methotrexate in patients with rheumatoid arthritis. *J Rheumatol* 21: 1224–1226

174 Worthley SG, McNeil JD (1995) Leukoencephalopathy in a patient taking low dose oral methotrexate therapy for rheumatoid arthritis. *J Rheumatol* 22: 335–337

175 Blackburn WDJ, Alarcón GS (1989) Impotence in three rheumatoid arthritis patients treated with methotrexate. *Arthritis Rheum* 32: 1341–1342

176 Del Paine DW, Leek JC, Robbins DL (1980) Gynecomastia associated with low dose methotrexate therapy. *Arthritis Rheum* 26: 691–692

177 Phelan MJ, Riley PL, Lynch MP (1992) Methotrexate associated Peyronie's disease in the treatment of rheumatoid arthritis. *Br J Rheumatol* 31: 425–426

178 Kozlowski RD, Steinbrunner JV, Mackenzie AH, Clough JD, Wilke WS, Segal AM (1990) Outcome of first-trimester exposure to low-dose methotrexate in eight patients with rheumatic disease. *Am J Med* 88: 589–592

179 Buckley LM, Bullaboy CA, Leichtman L, Marquez M (1997) Multiple congenital anomalies associated with weekly low-dose methotrexate treatment of the mother. *Arthritis Rheum* 40: 971–973

180 Centers for Disease Control (1992) Recommendations for the use of folic acid to reduce the number of cases of spina bifida and other neural tube defects. *MMWR (RR-14)* 1–7

181 Yetley EA, Rader JI (1995) Folate fortification of cereal grains: FDA policies and actions. *Cereal Foods World* 40:67-72

182 Schwartz AM, Leonidas JC (1984) Methotrexate osteopathy. *Skeletal Radiol* 11:13–16

183 Maenaut K, Westhovens R, Dequeker J (1996) Methotrexate osteopathy, does it exist? *J Rheumatol* 23: 2156–2159

184 Zonneveld IM, Bakker WK, Dijkstra PF, Bos JD, van Soesbergen RM, Dinant HJ (1996) Methotrexate osteopathy in long-term, low-dose methotrexate treatment for psoriasis and rheumatoid arthritis. *Archives Dermatol* 132: 184–187

185 Buckley LM, Leib ES, Cartularo KS, Vacek PM, Cooper SM (1997) Effect of low dose methotrexate on the bone mineral density of patients with rheumatoid arthritis. *J Rheumatol* 24: 1489–1494

186 May KP, West SG, McDermott MT, Huffer WE (1994) The effect of low-dose methotrexate on bone metabolism and histomorphometry in rats. *Arthritis Rheum* 37: 201–206

187 Halevy S, Giryes H, Avinoach I, Livni E, Sukenik S (1998) Leukocytoclastic vasculitis induced by low-dose methotrexate: *in vitro* evidence for an immunologic mechanism. *J Euro Acad Dermatol Venereol* 10: 81–85

188 Simonart T, Durez P, Margaux J, Van Geertruyden J, Goldschmidt D, Parent D (1997) Cutaneous necrotizing vasculitis after low dose methotrexate therapy for rheumatoid arthritis: a possible manifestation of methotrexate hypersensitivity. *Clin Rheumatol* 16: 623–625

189 Kaye O, Beckers CC, Paquet P, Arrese JE, Piérard GE, Malaise MG (1996) The frequency of cutaneous vasculitis is not increased in patients with rheumatoid arthritis treated with methotrexate. *J Rheumatol* 23: 253–257

190 Segal R, Caspi D, Tishler M, Fishel B, Yaron M (1988) Accelerated nodulosis and vasculitis during methotrexate therapy for rheumatoid arthritis. *Arthritis Rheum* 31: 1182–1185

191 Jeurissen MEC, Boerbooms AMT, van de Putte LBA (1989) Eruption of nodulosis and vasculitis during methotrexate therapy for rheumatoid arthritis. *Clin Rheumatol* 8: 417–418

192 Blackburn WDJ, Alarcón GS (1990) Toxic response to topical fluorouracil in two rheumatoid arthritis patients receiving low-dose, weekly methotrexate. *Arthritis Rheum* 33: 303–304

193 Falcini F, Taccetti G, Ernimi M, Trapani S, Calzolari A, Franchi A, Cerinic MM (1997) Methotrexate-associated appearance and rapid progression of rheumatoid nodules in systemic-onset juvenile rheumaotid arthritis. *Arthritis Rheum* 40: 175–178

194 Kerstens PJ, Boerbooms AM, Jeurissen ME, Fast JH, Assmann KJ, van de Putte LB (1992) Accelerated nodulosis during low dose methotrexate therapy for rheumatoid arthritis. An analysis of ten cases. *J Rheumatol* 19: 867–871

195 Smith MD (1995) Accelerated nodulosis, pleural effusion, and pericardial tamponade during methotrexate therapy. *J Rheumatol* 22: 1439

196 Abu-Shakra M, Nicol P, Urowitz MB (1994) Accelerated nodulosis, pleural effusion, and pericardial tamponade during methotrexate therapy. *J Rheumatol* 21: 934–937

197 Combe B, Didry C, Gutierrez M, Anaya JM, Sany J (1993) Accelerated nodulosis and systemic manifestations during methotrexate therapy for rheumatoid arthritis. *Eur J Med* 2: 153–156

198 Merrill JT, Shen C, Schreibman D, Coffey D, Zakharenko O, Fisher R, Lahita RG, Salmon J, Cronstein BN (1997) Adenosine A1 receptor promotion of multinucleated giant cell formation by human monocytes: a mechanism for methotrexate-induced nodulosis in rheumatoid arthritis. *Arthritis Rheum* 40: 1308–1315

199 Essig KM, Mayet WJ, Mottrie AM, Helmreich-Becker I, Meyer zum Buschenfelde KH (1994) Rheumatoid nodules located in the penis of a methotrexate-treated patient with rheumatoid arthritis. *Zeitschrift Rheumatol* 53: 314–316

200 Chatham WW (1992) Methotrexate associated rheumatoid nodulosis-improvement with addition of sulfasalazine (abstract). *Arthritis Rheum* 35: R15

201 Karam NE, Roger L, Hankins LL, Reveille JD (1994) Rheumatoid nodulosis of the meninges. *J Rheumatol* 21: 1960–1963

202 Raccaud O (1994) Manifestations extra-articulaires de la polyarthrite rheumatoide lors d'un traitement de fond par methotrexate: a propos d'un cas de nodulose avec pericardite. [Extra-articular manifestations of rheumatoid arthritis at the time of basic methotrexate treatment: apropos of a case of nodulosis with pericarditis]. *Rev Med Suisse Rom* 114: 343–344

203 Bruyn GA, Essed CE, Houtman PM, Willemse FW (1993) Fatal cardiac nodules in a patient with rheumatoid arthritis treated with low dose methotrexate. *J Rheumatol* 20: 912–914

204 Moder KG, Tefferi A, Cohen MD, Menke DM, Luthra HS (1995) Hematologic malignancies and the use of methotrexate in rheumatoid arthritis: a retrospective study. *Am J Med* 99: 276–281

205 Pointud P, Prudat M, Peron J (1993) Acute leukemia after low dose methotrexate therapy in a patient with rheumatoid arthritis. *J Rheumatol* 20: 1215–1216

206 Bologna C, Picot MC, Jorgensen C, Viu P, Verdier R, Sany J (1997) Study of eight cases of cancer in 426 rheumatoid arthritis patients treated with methotrexate. *Ann Rheum Dis* 56: 97–102

207 Kingsmore SF, Hall BD, Allen NB, Rice JR, Caldwell DS (1992) Association of methotrexate, rheumatoid arthritis and lymphoma: Report of 2 cases and literature review. *J Rheumatol* 19: 1462–1465

208 Thoburn R, Katz P (1995) Lymphoproliferative disease in patients with autoimmune disease on low-dose methotrexate. *Am Col Rheumatol Hotline* June:1

209 Georgescu L, Quinn GC, Schwartzman S, Paget SA (1997) Lymphoma in patients with rheumatoid arthritis: association with the disease state or methotrexate treatment. *Sem Arthritis Rheum* 26: 794–804

210 Usman AR, Yunus MB (1996) Non-Hodgkin's lymphoma in patients with rheumatoid arthritis treated with low dose methotrexate. *J Rheumatol* 23: 1095–1098

211 Bachman TR, Sawitzke AD, Perkins SL, Ward JH, Cannon GW (1996) Reversible lymphoma in rheumatoid arthritis patients treated with methotrexate: Report of two cases. *Arthritis Rheum* 39: 325–329

212 Thomason RW, Craig FE, Banks PM, Sears DL, Myerson GE, Gulley ML (1998) Epstein-Barr virus and lymphoproliferation in methotrexate-treated rheumatoid arthritis. *Modern Pathol* 9: 261–266

213 Salloum E, Cooper DL, Howe G, Lacy J, Tallini G, Crouch J, Schultz M, Murren J (1996) Spontaneous regression of lymphoproliferative disorders in patients treated with methotrexate for rheumatoid arthritis and other rheumatic diseases. *J Clin Oncol* 14: 1943–1949

214 Lioté F, Pertuiset E, Cochand-Priollet B, D'Agay M, Dombret H, Numéric P, D'Anglejan G, Kuntz D (1995) Methotrexate related B lymphoproliferative disease in a patient with rheumatoid arthritis. Role of Epstein-Barr virus infection. *J Rheumatol* 22: 1174–1178

215 Marlier S, Chagnon A, Brocq O, de Jaureguiberry JP, Jaubert D, Paris JF, Carli P (1995) Lymphoma induced by low-dose methotrexate in rheumatoid arthritis with severe lymphopenia. [Lymphome sous methotrexate a faibles doses au cours d'une polyarthrite rheumatoide avec lymphopenie extreme. *Ann Medic Intern* 146: 206–208

216 Ferraccioli GF, Casatta L, Bartoli E, De Vita S, Dolcetti R, Boiocchi M, Carbone A (1995) Epstein-Barr virus-associated Hodgkin's lymphoma in a rheumatoid arthritis patient treated with methotrexate and cyclosporin A. *Arthritis Rheum* 38: 867–868

217 Flipo RM, Delaporte E, Lecomte-Houcke M (1997) Cutaneous pseudolymphoma occurring during methotrexate therapy for rheumatoid arthritis. *J Rheumatol* 24: 809–810

218 Zimmer-Galler I, Lie JT (1994) Choroidal infiltrates as the initial manifestation of lymphoma in rheumatoid arthritis after treatment with low-dose methotrexate. *Mayo Clin Proc* 69: 258–261

219 Kamel OW, van de Rijn M, LeBrun DP, Weiss LM, Warnke RA, Dorfman RF (1994) Lymphoid neoplasms in patients with rheumatoid arthritis and dermatomyositis: fre-

quency of Epstein-Barr virus and other features associated with immunosuppression. *Human Pathol* 25: 638–643

220 Taillan B, Garnier G, Castanet J, Ferrari E, Pesce A, Dujardin P (1993) Lymphoma developing in a patient with rheumatoid arthritis taking methotrexate. *Clin Rheumatol* 12: 93–94

221 Kamel OW, van de Rijn M, Weiss LM, Del Zoppo GJ, Hench PK, Robbins BA, Montgomery PG, Warnke RA, Dorfman RF (1993) Brief report: Reversible lymphomas associated with Epstein-Barr virus occurring during methotrexate therapy for rheumatoid arthritis and dermatomyositis. *N Engl J Med* 328: 1317–1321

222 Barger BO, Acton RT, Koopman WJ, Alarcón GS (1984) DR antigens and gold toxicity in white rheumatoid arthritis patients. *Arthritis Rheum* 27: 601–605

223 Ellman MH, Hurwitz H, Thomas C, Kozloff M (1991) Lymphoma developing in a patient with rheumatoid arthritis taking low dose weekly methotrexate. *J Rheumatol* 18: 1741–1743

224 Le Goff P, Koreichi A, Saraux A, Baron A (1994) Lymphome au cours du traitement de la polyarthrite rhumatoide par le methotrexate a faible dose: un nouveau cas. [Lymphoma during treatment of rheumatoid arthritis with low-dose methotrexate: a new case]. *Rev Rheuma* 61: 357–358

225 Morris CR, Morris AJ (1993) Localized lymphoma in a patient with rheumatoid arthritis treated with parenteral methotrexate. *J Rheumatol* 20: 2172–2173

226 Padeh S, Sharon N, Schiby G, Rechavi G, Passwell JH (1997) Hodgkin's lymphoma in systemic onset juvenile rheumatoid arthritis after treatment with low dose methotrexate. *J Rheumatol* 24: 2035–2037

227 Boerbooms AM, Kerstens PJ, van Loenhout JW, Mulder J, van de Putte LB (1995) Infections during low-dose methotrexate treatment in rheumatoid arthritis. *Sem Arthritis Rheum* 24: 411–421

228 Van der Veen MJ, van der Heide A, Kruize AA, Bijisma JW (1994) Infection rate and use of antibiotics in patients with rheumatoid arthritis treated with methotrexate. *Ann Rheum Dis* 53: 224–228

229 Kanik KS, Cash JM (1997) Does methotrexate increase the risk of infection or malignancy. *Rheum Dis Clin N Am* 23: 955–967

230 Shiroky JB, Frost A, Skeleton JD, Haegert DG, Newkirk MM, Neville C (1991) Complications of immunosuppression associated with weekly low dose methotrexate. *J Rheumatol* 18: 1172–1175

231 Martinez-Osuna P, Zwolinska JB, Sikes DH, Cory JG, Silveira LH, Jara LJ, Espinoza LR (1993) Lack of immunosuppressive effect of low-dose oral methotrexate on lymphocytes in rheumatoid arthritis. *Clin Exper Rheumatol* 11: 249–253

232 Johnston CA, Russell AS, Kovithavongs T, Dasgupta M (1986) Measures of immunologic and inflammatory responses *in vitro* in rheumatoid patients treated with methotrexate. *J Rheumatol* 13: 294–296

233 Johnston C, Russell AS, Aaron S (1988) The effect of *in vivo* and *in vitro* methotrexate on lymphocyte proliferation as measured by the uptake of tritiated thymidine and tritiated guanosine. *Clin Exp Rheumatol* 6: 391–393

234 Hine RJ, Everson MP, Hardin JM, Morgan SL, Alarcón GS, Baggott JE, Koopman WJ, Krumdieck CL (1990) Methotrexate therapy in rheumatoid arthritis patients diminishes lectin-induced mononuclear cell proliferation. *Rheumatol Int* 10: 165–169

235 Olsen NJ, Murray LM (1989) Antiproliferative effects of methotrexate on peripheral blood mononuclear cells. *Arthritis Rheum* 32: 378–385

236 Olsen NJ, Callahan LF, Pincus T (1987) Immunologic studies of rheumatoid arthritis patients treated with methotrexate. *Arthritis Rheum* 30: 481–488

237 Lyon CC, Thompson D (1997) Herpes zoster encephalomyelitis associated with low dose methotrexate for rheumatoid arthritis. *J Rheumatol* 24: 589–591

238 Golden HE (1998) Herpes zoster encephalomyelitis in a patient with rheumatoid arthritis treated with low dose methotrexate. *J Rheumatol* 24: 2487–2488

239 Thomas E, Olive P, Mazyad H, Blotman F (1997) Cytomegalovirus-induced pneumonia in a rheumatoid arthritis patient treated with low dose methotrexate. *Clin Exp Rheumatol* 15: 583–584

240 Naides SJ (1995) Acute parvovirus B19-induced pancytopenia in the setting of methotrexate therapy for rheumatoid arthritis. *Arthritis Rheum* 38: 1023

241 McCambridge NM, Vogelgesang SA, Ockenhouse CF (1995) Listeria monocytogenes infection in a patient treated with methotrexate for rheumatoid arthritis. *J Rheumatol* 22: 786–787

242 Ching DW (1995) Severe, disseminated, life threatening herpes zoster infection in a patient with rheumatoid arthritis treated with methotrexate. *Ann Rheum Dis* 54: 155

243 Stenger AA, Houtman PM, Bruyn GA, Eggink HF, Pasma HR (1994) Pneumocystis carinii pneumonia associated with low dose methotrexate treatment for rheumatoid arthritis. *Scand J Rheumatol* 23: 51–53

244 O'Reilly S, Hartley P, Jeffers M, Casey E, Clancy L (1994) Invasive pulmonary aspergillosis associated with low dose methotrexate therapy for rheumatoid arthritis: a case report of treatment with itraconazole. *Tubercle Lung Dis* 75: 153–155

245 Perez T, D'Ansin E, Wallaert B, Tonnel AB (1991) [Pleuro-pulmonary manifestations of rheumatoid polyarthritis]. Manifestations pleuro-pulmonaries de la polyarthrite rheumatoide. *Rev Malad Respir* 8: 169–189

246 LeMense GP, Sahn SA (1994) Opportunistic infection during treatment with low dose methotrexate. *Am J Resp Crit Care Med* 150: 258–260

247 Wyss E, Kuhn M, Luzi HP, Reinhart WH (1994) Fatal verlaufende pneumocystis-carinii-pneumonie unter low-dose-methotrexat- und prednison-therapie wegen chronischer polyarthritis. [Fatal outcome of pneumocystis-carinii pneumonia under low-dose methotrexate and prednisone therapy for chronic rheumatoid arthritis]. *Schweiz Rundsch Med Prax* 83: 449–452

248 Lang B, Riegel W, Peters T, Peter HH (1991) Low dose methotrexate therapy for rheumatoid arthritis complicated by pancytopenia and pneumocystis carinii pneumonia. *J Rheumatol* 18: 1257–1259

249 Flood DA, Chan CK, Pruzanski W (1991) Pneumocystis carinii pneumonia associated with methotrexate therapy in rheumatoid arthritis. *J Rheumatol* 18: 1254–1256

250 Cornelissen JJ, Bakker LJ, Van der Veen MJ, Rozenberg-Arska M, Bijlsma JW (1991) *Nocardia asteroides* pneumonia complicating low dose methotrexate treatment of refractory rheumatoid arthritis. *Ann Rheum Dis* 50: 642–644

251 Wollner AA, Mohle-Boetani J, Lambert RE, Perruquet JL, Raffin TA, McGuire JL (1991) Pneumocystis carinii pneumonia complicating low dose methotrexate treatment for rheumatoid arthritis. *Thorax* 46: 205–207

252 Antonelli MA, Moreland LW, Brick JE (1991) Herpes zoster in patients with rheumatoid arthritis treated with weekly, low-dose methotrexate. *Am J Med* 90: 295–298

253 Aspe de la Iglesia B, Sanchez Burson, Grana Gil, Galdo Fernandez F (1990) Pancytopenia and opportunistic infections in rheumatoid arthritis treated with methotrexate. [Pancitopenia e infecciones oportunistas en artritis reumatoid tratada con metotrexato]. *Rev Clin Espanol* 187: 208–209

254 Altz-Smith M, Kendall LGJ, Stamm AM (1987) Cryptococcosis associated with low-dose methotrexate for arthritis. *Am J Med* 83: 179–181

255 Perruquet JL, Harrington TM, Davis DE (1983) *Pneumocystis carinii* pneumonia following methotrexate therapy for rheumatoid arthritis. *Arthritis Rheum* 26: 1291–1292

256 Bridges SL Jr, Moreland LW (1997) Perioperative use of methotrexate in patients with rheumatoid arthritis undergoing orthopedic surgery. *Rheum Dis Clin N Am* 23: 981–993

257 Steuer A, Keat AC (1998) Perioperative use of methotrexate – a survey of clinical practice in the United Kingdom. *Br J Rheumatol* 36: 1009–1011

258 Carpenter MT, West SG, Vogelgesang SA, Jones DEC (1996) Postoperative joint infections in rheumatoid arthritis patients on methotrexate therapy. *Orthopedics* 19: 207–210

259 Escalante A, Beardmore TD (1998) Risk factors for early wound complications after orthopedic surgery for rheumatoid arthritis. *J Rheumatol* 22: 1844–1851

260 Kasdan ML, June L (1993) Postoperative results of rheumatoid arthritis patients on methotrexate at the time of reconstructive surgery of the hand. *Orthopedics* 16: 1233–1235

261 Sany J, Anaya J, Canovas F, Combe B, Jorgensen C, Saker S, Thaury MN, Gavroy JP (1993) Influence of methotrexate on the frequency of postoperative infectious complications in patients with rheumatoid arthritis. *J Rheumatol* 20: 1129–1132

262 Bridges SLJ, López-Méndez A, Han KH, Tracy IC, Alarcón GS (1991) Should methotrexate be discontinued before elective orthopedic surgery in patients with rheumatoid arthritis? *J Rheumatol* 18: 984–988

263 Perhala RS, Wilke WS, Clough JD, Segal AM (1991) Local infectious complications fol-
    lowing large joint replacement in rheumatoid arthritis patients treated with methotrexate
    vs. those not treated with methotrexate. *Arthritis Rheum* 34: 146–152
264 Alarcón GS, Moreland LW, Jaffe K, Mikhail I, Phillips M, Bocanegra TS, Russell J (1995)
    Barriers encountered in the conduct of clinical studies: A case in point. Perioperatively dis-
    continuation of methotrexate. *Controlled Clin Trials* 16: 122S
265 Jundt JW, Browne BA, Fiocco GP, Steele AD, Mock D (1993) A comparison of low dose
    methotrexate bioavailability: oral solution, oral tablet, subcutaneous and intramuscular
    dosing. *J Rheumatol* 20: 1845–1849
266 Brooks PJ, Spruill WJ, Parish RC, Birchmore DA (1990) Pharmacokinetics of metho-
    trexate administered by intramuscular and subcutaneous injections in patients with
    rheumatoid arthritis. *Arthritis Rheum* 33: 91–94
267 Gertner E, Marshall PS (1996) Oral administration of an easily prepared solution of in-
    jectable methotrexate diluted in water: A comparison of serum concentrations vs.
    methotrexate tablets and clinical utility. *J Rheumatol* 23: 455–458
268 Hamilton RA, Kremer JM (1997) Why intramuscular methotrexate may be more ef-
    ficacious than oral dosing in patients with rheumatoid arthritis. *Br J Rheumatol* 36: 86–90
269 Franchi F, Seminara P, Codacci-Pisanelli G, Aronne T, Avella A, Bonomo L (1989)
    Intrarticular methotrexate in the therapy of rheumatoid arthritis. *Rec Progressi Med* 80:
    261–262
270 Hall GH, Jones BJ, Head AC, Jones VE (1978) Intra-articular methotrexate. Clinical and
    laboratory study in rheumatoid and psoriatic arthritis. *Ann Rheum Dis* 37: 351–356
271 Wigginton SM, Chu BCF, Weisman MH, Howell SB (1980) Methotrexate pharmacokine-
    tics after intraarticular injection in patients with rheumatoid arthritis. *Arthritis Rheum* 23:
    119–122
272 Furst DE, Koehnke R, Burmeister LF, Kohler J, Cargill I (1989) Increasing methotrexate
    effect with increasing dose in the treatment of resistant rheumatoid arthritis. *J Rheumatol*
    16: 313–320
273 Schnabel A, Reinhold-Keller E, Willmann V, Gross WL (1994) Tolerability of metho-
    trexate starting with 15 or 25 mg/week for rheumatoid arthritis. *Rheumatol Int* 14: 33–38
274 Kozloski GD, De Vito J, Kisicki JC, Johnson JB (1992) The effect of food on the absorp-
    tion of methotrexate sodium tablets in healthy volunteers. *Arthritis Rheum* 35: 761–764
275 Oguey D, Kolliker F, Gerber NJ, Reichen J (1992) Effect of food on the bioavailability of
    low-dose methotrexate in patients with rheumatoid arthritis. *Arthritis Rheum* 35: 611–614
276 American College of Rheumatology AD HOC Committee in Clinical Guidelines. (1996)
    Guidelines for monitoring drug therapy in rheumatoid arthritis. *Arthritis Rheum* 39:
    723–731
277 Tishler M, Caspi D, Fishel B, Yaron M (1988) The effects of leucovorin (folinic acid) on
    methotrexate therapy in rheumatoid arthritis patients. *Arthritis Rheum* 31: 906–908
278 Weinblatt ME, Maier AL, Coblyn JS (1993) Low dose leucovorin does not interfere with
    the efficacy of methotrexate in rheumatoid arthritis: An 8 week randomized placebo con-
    trolled trial. *J Rheumatol* 20: 950–952
279 Hanrahan PS, Russell AS (1988) Concurrent use of folinic acid and methotrexate in rheu-
    matoid arthritis. *J Rheumatol* 15: 1078–1080
280 Shiroky JB, Neville C, Esdaile JM, Choquette D, Zummer M, Hazeltine M, Bykerk V,
    Kanji M, St-Pierre A, Robidoux L, et al (1993) Low-dose methotrexate with leucovorin
    (folinic acid) in the management of rheumatoid arthritis. Results of a multicenter
    randomized, double-blinded, placebo-controlled trial. *Arthritis Rheum* 36: 795–803
281 Hunt RE, Phillips RM, Shergy WJ (1987) Role of folic acid in limiting methotrexate
    related side effects. *Arthritis Rheum* 30: S253 (Abstract)
282 Ortiz Z, Shea B, Suarez-Almazor M, Moher D, Wells G, Tugwell P (1998) The efficacy of
    folic acid and folinic acid in reducing methotrexate side effects in rheumatoid arthritis. A
    meta-analysis of randomized controlled trials. *J Rheumatol* 25: 36–43
283 Grecomoro G, Piccione F, Letizia G (1992) Therapeutic synergism between hyaluronic
    acid and dexamethasone in the intra-articular treatment of osteoarthritis of the knee: A
    preliminary open study. *Curr Med Res Opin* 13: 49–55
284 Morgan SL, Baggott JE, Alarcón GS, Koopman WJ, Krumdieck CL (1994) Leucovorin vs.
    folic acid in the treatment of methotrexate toxicity: comment on the article by Shiroky et
    al. *Arthritis Rheum* 37: 444

285 Harris ED Jr (1990) Rheumatoid arthritis: Pathophysiology and implications for therapy. *N Engl J Med* 322: 1277–1289

286 Harris ED Jr (1995) Treatment of rheumatoid arthritis ... for now and the future. In: Kelley WN, Harris ED Jr, Ruddy S, Sledge CB (ed): *Textbook of Rheumatology.* W.B. Saunders Company, New York, 1–20

287 O'Dell JR (1997) Methotrexate use in rheumatoid arthritis. *Rheum Dis Clin N Am* 23: 779–796

288 Collins D, Bellamy N, Campbell J (1994) A Canadian survey of current methotrexate prescribing practices in rheumatoid arthritis. *J Rheumatol* 21: 1220–1223

289 Galindo-Rodriguez G, Avina-Zubieta JA, Fitzgerald A, LeClerq SA, Russell AS, Suarez-Almazor ME (1997) Variations and trends in the prescription of initial second line therapy for patients with rheumatoid arthritis. *J Rheumatol* 24: 633–638

290 Suarez-Almazor ME, Soskolne CL, Saunders LD, Russell AS (1995) Use of second line drugs for the treatment of rheumatoid arthritis in Edmonton, Alberta. Patterns of prescription and longterm effectiveness. *J Rheumatol* 22: 836–843

291 Sostman HD, Matthay RA, Putman CE, Smith GJW (1976) Methotrexate-induced pneumonitis. *Medicine* 55: 371–388

292 Haagsma CJ, Russel FGM, Vree TB, van Riel PLCM, van de Putte LBA (1996) Combination of methotrexate and sulphasalazine in patients with rheumatoid arthritis: pharmacokinetic analysis and relationship to clinical response. *Br J Clin Pharmacol* 42: 195–200

293 Boers M, Verhoeven AC, Markusse HM, van de Laar AFJ, Westhovens R, van Denderen JC, van Zeben D, Dijkmans BAC, Peeters AJ, Jacobs P, et al (1997) Randomised comparison of combined step-down prednisolone, methotrexate and sulphasalazine with sulphasalazine alone in early rheumatoid arthritis. *Lancet* 350: 309–318

294 Haagsma CJ, van Riel PL, de Jong AJ, van de Putte LB (1997) Combination of sulphasalazine and methotrexate vs. the single components in early rheumatoid arthritis: a randomized, controlled, double-blind, 52 week clinical trial. *Br J Rheumatol* 36: 1082–1088

295 O'Dell JR, Haire CE, Erikson N, Drymalski W, Palmer W, Eckhoff PJ, Garwood V, Maloley P, Klassen LW, Wees S, et al (1996) Treatment of rheumatoid arthritis with methotrexate alone, sulfasalazine and hydroxychloroquine, or a combination of all three medications. *N Engl J Med* 334: 1287–1291

296 Ferraz MB, Pinheiro GR, Helfenstein M, Albuquerque E, Rezende C, Roimicher L, Brandao L, Silva SC, Pinheiro GC, Atra E (1994) Combination therapy with methotrexate and chloroquine in rheumatoid arthritis. A multicenter randomized placebo-controlled trial. *Scand J Rheumatol* 23: 231–236

297 Willkens RF, Stablein D (1996) Combination treatment of rheumatoid arthiritis using azathioprine and methotrexate: A 48 week controlled clinical trial. *J Rheumatol* 23: 64–68

298 Willkens RF, Sharp JT, Stablein D, Marks C, Wortmann R (1995) Comparison of azathioprine, methotrexate, and the combination of the two in the treatment of rheumatoid arthritis: A forty-eight-week controlled clinical trial with radiologic outcome assessment. *Arthritis Rheum* 38: 1799–1806

299 Stein CM, Pincus T, Yocum D, Tugwell P, Wells G, Gluck O, Kraag G, Torley H, Tesser J, McKendry R, et al (1997) Combination treatment of severe rheuatoid arthritis with cyclosporine and methotrexate for forty-eight weeks. An open-label extension study. *Arthritis Rheum* 40: 1843–1851

300 Stein CM, Brooks RH, Pincus T (1997) Effect of combination therapy with cyclosporine and methotrexate on liver function test results in rheumatoid arthritis. *Arthritis Rheum* 40: 1721–1723

301 Tugwell P, Pincus T, Yocum D, Stein M, Gluck O, Kraag G, McKendry R, Tesser J, Baker P, Wells G, et al (1995) Combination therapy with cyclosporine and methotrexate in severe rheumatoid arthritis. *N Engl J Med* 333: 137–141

302 Rozman B, for the Leflunomide Investigators' Group (1998) Clinical experience with leflunomide in rheumatoid arthritis. *J Rheumatol* 25: 27–32

303 Kitsuwa S, Matsunaga K, Kawai M, Tsuzi T, Kato K, Tani K, Okubo T (1996) Pancytopenia and pneumocystis carinii pneumonia associated with low dose methotrexate pulse therapy for rheumatoid arthritis-case report and review of literature. *Ryumachi* 36: 551–558

304 Okuda Y, Oyama T, Oyama H, Miyamoto T, Takasugi K (1995) Pneumocystis carinii
      pneumonia associated with low dose methotrexate treatment for malignant rheumatoid
      arthritis. *Ryumachi* 35: 699–704
305 Espinoza LR, Espinoza CG, Vasey FB, Germain BF (1986) Oral methotrexate therapy for
      chronic rheumatoid arthritis ulcerations. *J Am Acad Dermatol* 15: 508–512
306 Olivieri I, Salvarani C, Cantini F (1997) Remitting distal extremity swelling with pitting
      edema: a distinct syndrome or a clinical feature of different inflammatory rheumatic
      diseases? *J Rheumatol* 224: 249–252
307 Kamper AM, Malbrain M, Zachee P, Chew SL (1994) Parvovirus infection causing red cell
      aplasia and leukopenia in rheumatoid arthritis. *Clin Rheumatol* 13: 129–131

Methotrexate
ed. by B. N. Cronstein und J. R. Bertino
© 2000 Birkhäuser Verlag Basel/Switzerland

Use of methotrexate in the treatment of psoriasis and other dermatological disorders

Charles McDonald

Department of Dermatology, Rhode Island Hospital/Brown University, 593 Eddy St., Providence, RI 02903, USA

Introduction

Following the demonstration by Rees et al. that the skin disease psoriasis is quite often responsive to treatment with methotrexate (MTX) other investigators began to examine its use in a wide variety of benign and malignant cutaneous diseases [1–6] (Tab. 1). Most of these diseases have been shown to arise as a result of severe inflammation, cellular hyperproliferation, tissue hyperplasia, or a combination of these. Because psoriasis is the most common of this group of diseases, estimated to occur in 1–2% of western European populations [7], much of the discussion on the use of MTX in skin disease will be given to MTX and its use in psoriasis.

Table 1. Skin diseases in which methotrexate has been found useful

Hyperproliferative	– Psoriasis and psoriatic arthritis – Pityriasis rubra pilaris – Epidermolytic hyperkeratosis – Lamellar ichthyosis
Malignancies	– Cutaneous T-cell lymphoma (mycosis fungoides and Sézary's syndrome)
Vasculitis	– Polyarteritis nodosa (cutaneous and systemic) – Wegener's granulomatosis
Systemic connective tissue diseases	– Dermatomyositis
Bullous diseases	– Pemphigus – Pemphigoid
Inflammatory skin diseases	– Pityriasis lichenoides et varioliformis (Mucha-Habermann disease) – Sarcoidosis

Psoriasis

Introduction

Multiple factors influence the onset and course of psoriasis. Among these are heredity, environment, psyche, physical trauma, emotional trauma, and abnormal inflammation. Based on inheritance, psoriasis patients are often divided into two groups: Type I in which psoriasis has an early onset associated with a strong family history and an associated HLA-CW6 genotype; and Type II in which psoriasis has its onset late in life and has little or no association with the HLA-CW6 genotype. Type I tends toward an unrelenting and unfavorable outcome. Each of these associations have been found most commonly in northern Europeans.

Clinically, psoriasis presents as isolated, or clusters of red, scaling papules that coalesce to form plaques. The nature of the disease is such that it enters periods of extreme activity followed by periods of complete quiescence. Trauma to the skin is sometimes followed by the appearance of typical psoriatic papules and plaques (the Koebner isomorphic response). A wide variety of acute infectious diseases may be followed by the appearance of scattered "drop-like" or guttate lesions. This is particularly true of disease occurring after group A streptococcal infections.

Psoriasis may also occur in pustular forms in the absence of any associated or causative bacteria. Localized pustular disease, principally found on the palms and soles or around inflamed joints of the digits, is most commonly observed. Generalized pustular disease may occur secondary to the withdrawal of systemic corticosteroids, after extensive topical corticosteroid use, or following generalized drug eruptions. Psoriasis involving the entire integument may also result in erythrodermic disease, often indistinguishable from erythroderma caused by other diseases.

Arthritis may be found in up to 25% of patients with psoriasis. Its onset often precedes the appearance of psoriasis by many years, or it may begin many years after the onset of psoriasis. Psoriatic arthritis characteristically involves the distal interphalangeal joints of the hands and feet, as well as larger joints of the wrist and the sacroilium. A negative test for rheumatoid factor is found in this disease. In any single patient arthritis may progress slowly or rapidly, occasionally ending in severe arthritis mutilans.

Pathology

The histopathological picture in early stage psoriasis is often not characteristic. Parakeratosis may occur and lymphocytes and macrophages may be seen invading the epidermis. A moderate infiltration of lymphocytes and macrophages in the papillary dermis may be all that is seen. There may also be dilatation of capillaries and edema within the dermal papillae. In a mature psoriasis plaque characteristic pathology is seen. There is thickening of the epidermis due to overall elongation of the rete ridges and a compensatory elongation of the dermal papillae. The rete ridges are also bulbous at the base. Thinning of the supra-papillary portion of the epidermis, absence of a granular layer in the epidermis, parakeratosis, and the presence of microabscess within the epidermis are seen. The number of mitoses per unit surface area is increased. Dermal capillaries are dilated and tortuous. There is a monomorphous inflammatory infiltrate surrounding dermal blood vessels. The number of inflammatory cells within the epidermis increases to the extent that microcollections of leukocytic cells will produce microscopic intraepidermal clusters, many containing neutrophils.

Etiology and pathogenesis

Psoriasis is a disease in which multiple defects are found within the epidermis and dermis. Within the epidermis, psoriasis is characterized by increased cellular proliferation of epidermal keratinocytes and accelerated and incomplete epidermal cell differentiation [8]. The ultimate outcome is a marked scaling and shedding of the involved skin. Dermal disease is characterized by inflammation and the presence of abnormal cutaneous vasculature [9, 10]. Dermal disease is associated with extravasation of monocytes, lymphocytes, and neutrophils into the dermis and enhancement of infiltrates of neutrophils and activated T lymphocytes throughout the epidermis and dermis. Neutrophils within the epidermis often form microscopic abscesses, particularly within the subcorneal layer of the epidermis. Macrocollections may also occur, resulting in macroabscesses or the typical clinical lesions observed in pustular psoriasis. Directed leukocyte migration to epidermis appears to be due in part to altered leukocyte extracellular matrix interactions [11]. In active psoriasis peripheral blood leukocytes show decreased adherence to extracellular dermal components, especially those of the basement membrane, as collagen types I and IV, laminin, and fibronectin.

Helper T-lymphocytes play a very active role in the pathogenesis of psoriasis. Lymphocytes within the epidermis and dermis are primarily of two types: CD4$^+$ (75%) and CD8$^+$ (25%) (12). Activation of T lymphocytes precedes epidermal proliferation. The percentage of CD4$^+$ versus CD8$^+$ cells varies in chronic and acute disease.

Some laboratory investigations suggest a number of possibilities relative to the pathogenesis of psoriasis. The chronic phase of psoriasis appears to be very active immunologically and is possibly more active than during early onset disease. CD4$^+$ cells, through the production of active cytokines, play an important role in the early onset of psoriasis. In late stage disease the role of CD4$^+$ cells may be lessened to be assumed by active CD8$^+$ cells.

Activated T cells produce a variety of regulatory cytokines such as IL-2, IFN-γ, and TNF (tumor necrosis factor). In addition to their active participation in the inflammatory process, some cytokines may stimulate proliferation of epidermal keratinocytes. It is also suggested that E-selectin and VCAM-1 expression on endothelial cells of the papillary microvessels may be critical for the initial trafficking of memory T cells and other cell types into psoriatic lesions. There is also a suggestion that the lymphocyte function-associated antigen-1α/ICAM-1 pathway may play an important role with regard to cell adhesion of infiltrating cells in psoriasis during disease exacerbation or prolongation.

Other investigations into the pathogenesis of psoriasis have shown that activated keratinocytes of the epidermis have the ability to synthesize and release a variety of cytokines such as IL-1 and IL-6, and granulocyte-macrophage colony simulating factor (GM-CSF), which can stimulate local T-cell activation [13, 14]. Locally activated T cells expressing such markers as high levels of major histocompatibility complex (MCH) class IV molecules and CD25 (IL-2 receptors), may be attracted to, and recruit other inflammatory cells that ultimately infiltrate, the epidermis thus accounting for the presence of inflammatory infiltrates in great quantities within the epidermis. Local triggering of activated T cells within the skin may lead to additional proliferation and biochemical activation of epidermal keratinocytes through ordinary cytokine pathways in a process very much like that which occurs in an activated cellular immune reaction.

The variety of abnormalities found in psoriasis, as inflammation, cellular hyperproliferation, and autoimmune T-cell and cytokine activation, make it difficult to pinpoint a specific metabolic site or sites for the action of MTX. It is most likely that MTX affects a number of metabolic sites in this disease. A number of investigators have concluded that biochemical events that occur in an active plaque of psoriasis serve as evidence that psoriasis is primarily an epidermal disease in which keratinocyte activation precedes any other alterations, and that epidermal activation triggers local inflammation [15].

Indications for use of methotrexate in psoriasis

The majority of patients with psoriasis can be effectively treated with the large variety of topical agents that are available over-the-counter or by prescription. In the treatment of psoriasis it should be remembered that most patients will experience periodic episodes of clearing, alternating with periods of disease exacerbation. Based on extensive clinical experience it is estimated that only 5–10% of patients with psoriasis will require at some time treatment with immunomodulatory and cytotoxic drugs. Immunomodulatory and cytotoxic drugs should be reserved for patients who have undergone appropriate intensive and extensive treatment with topical agents and regimens, and have failed to show evidence of clinical response, have experienced some adverse event during such treatment, or have experienced rapidly recurring bouts of disease after successful treatment. In general, these patients should have extensive and debilitating disease or have disease that impairs the performance of normal daily activities, that is, it affects the patient's economic, psychosocial, or physical well being. Table 2 describes such patients. For example, the latter group may include a salesperson or a nurse with severe hand psoriasis who is expected to use or expose his/her hands while carrying out assigned tasks. In these circumstances, severely affected psoriatic hands may be repulsive to customers of the salesperson, or may not permit the nurse to perform routine "scrubs" without adversely affecting the status of his/her psoriasis.

Table 2. Indication for use of methotrexate in benign cutaneous disease

Disease	Indications
Psoriasis	– Psoriasis of any type that is refractory to commonly used topical treatment. – Erythrodermic psoriasis – Photosensitive psoriasis – Pustular psoriasis, localized and generalized – Psoriasis that jeopardizes economic, psychosocial, or physical well being.
Dermatomyositis	– Disease that is non-responsive to corticosteroids in high dosages – Disease that requires prolonged high dosages of corticosteroids for maintenance (steroid sparing). – Patients with diseases that may be aggravated by high dose of corticosteroids, i.e. diabetes, hypertension, etc.
Polyarteritis nodosa and Wegener's granulomatosis	– Disease that does not respond to corticosteroids – Disease that requires prolonged high dosages of corticosteroids for maintenance (steroid sparing). – Patients with diseases that may be aggravated by high doses of corticosteroids, i.e. diabetes, hypertension, etc
Cutaneous T-cell lymphoma	– Cutaneous disease that is non-responsive to commonly used topical agents and modalities – Disease that has become systemic
Bullous diseases	– Disease refractory to corticosteroids – Disease that requires high dose, prolonged use of corticosteroids for maintenance of control (steroid sparing).
Pityriasis rubra pilaris	– Patients with diseases that may be aggravated by high doses of corticosteroids for disease control.
Sarcoidosis	– Disease non-responsive to corticosteroids. – Disease that requires prolonged use of high dosages of corticosteroids (steroid sparing).

Method of treatment of psoriasis

Each physician who is called upon to treat patients with psoriasis should develop a plan or a series of plans that can be engaged when patients present with one of the myriad varieties of psoriasis. Localized plaque psoriasis requires a different regimen versus that used for extensive plaque disease, or pustular psoriasis of the localized or generalized type, or guttate psoriasis, or erythrodermic psoriasis.

Failure of a psoriasis patient to respond to intensive topical agents and regimens should lead one to consider the use of systemic therapy.

Today MTX is considered the "gold standard" for systemic treatment of severe recalcitrant psoriasis. It is quite effective in controlling most forms of severe psoriasis and is quite safe in the properly monitored patient. There are very few contraindications to the use of MTX (Tab. 3). Among these are known liver disease, severely compromised renal function, severe hematological disease, severe systemic infections and, most importantly, an unreliable patient. Caution must be exercised in administering this agent to persons addicted to alcohol, to the elderly, who are often folic acid deficient and have poor renal function, and to females of childbearing age.

The pretreatment evaluation of a patient who is being considered for MTX is seen in (Tab. 4). It begins with a good history and physical examination to assess the patient's competence, emotional stability, and general medical status. A good history will also identify illnesses and medications that may potentiate or interfere with the metabolism of MTX. Standard

Table 3. Contraindications to the use of methotrexate in psoriasis

- Patients with known liver disease
- Patients with severely compromised renal function
- Patients with severe hematological disease
- Patients with severe systemic infections
- Females of childbearing age who are not practicing birth control
- Patients with known excessive alcohol consumption
- An unreliable patient
- Caution should be exercised in the elderly, diabetic and obese

Table 4. Pretreatment evaluation for use of methotrexate in psoriasis

- Complete history and physical examination
- Complete blood count including platelets
- Test of renal function blood urea nitrogen (BUN) and creatinine; and creatinine clearance in the elderly
- Liver function tests
- Serum chemistries
- Liver biopsy
- Chest x-ray
- Serum folate and B-12 in elderly patients

laboratory examinations prior to treatment include a complete blood count, measures of kidney and liver function, a chest x-ray and, in the elderly, a measure of serum folate and B12 levels should be done.

At least 10–20% of patients who submit to liver biopsies will show some form of liver abnormality. Additionally, it appears that patients who are obese, diabetic or consume large quantities of alcohol are quite prone to developing a type of liver disease often described as MTX-induced liver disease. Therefore, a liver biopsy is a requirement at or very near the beginning of treatment. It is needed as a baseline indicator for the presence or absence of antecedent liver disease. There should be very few exceptions to this policy. Treatment of psoriasis with MTX is a very serious undertaking and should be approached in a serious manner. The exception to performing pretreatment biopsy is a patient over 75 years of age whose life expectancy is such that an accumulative MTX toxic liver effect will not likely be reached. A total dosage of MTX above 1,500 mg is normally administered before measurable pathological disease may be experienced. The therapist should be aware of pretreatment liver defects so that he/she, if electing to initiate or continue MTX, will be able to devise a treatment regimen that will include a repeat liver biopsy prior to reaching the standard total dosage ordinarily recommended for posttreatment liver biopsy. The latent discovery of typical psoriasis-MTX liver disease in a patient who has taken MTX, and has not previously submitted to a pretreatment biopsy places the therapist at considerable risk in our litigious society. The patient who submits to pretreatment liver biopsy is clearly being informed of the seriousness of the treatment regimen he/she is about to undertake. Lastly, experience has shown it is quite rare to find a patient with severe psoriasis who does not tolerate MTX.

Monitoring

A good program of monitoring each patient for the appearance of toxic drug effects should be established (Tab. 5). A good monitoring program is the best insurance for the safe and effective use of MTX in cutaneous disease.

A complete blood count with platelets is repeated at appropriate intervals prior to the patient receiving MTX. A low white cell or platelet count calls for a temporary cessation of treatment until the count(s) returns to a normal level. It has been recommended that even in the absence of abnormal liver function tests, which should be repeated quarterly, a repeat liver biopsy should be done after an accumulative MTX dosage of 1,500 mg. Further biopsies will depend on the nature of the histopathological findings at biopsy. Some therapists have continued MTX after finding overt liver disease on liver biopsy and report no progression of the disease. In these patients, liver changes have been noted to return to normal after discontinuing alcohol and while continuing to receive MTX [16].

Table 5. Methotrexate monitoring guidelines

- Complete blood count with platelets, weekly, just prior to the administration of drug (in the long-term patient this schedule may be modified). A low platelet or white cell (WBC) count necessitates withholding of drug until the blood count returns to normal. Repeat folate and B12 are done if low WBC persists.[a]
- Chemistry profile to include liver function studies is done every 3–4 months, and at least 7 days after the last dose of MTX. Abnormal liver function studies should be repeated. If abnormal after 3 consecutive months of testing the liver biopsy is repeated.
- Repeat liver biopsy is done after a cumulative dosage of 1.5 g has been reached. This timing may vary based on each center's experience.
- If evidence of cirrhosis is found liver biopsy should be repeated after 1 year.
- Increased severity of cirrhosis on repeat liver biopsy requires discontinuing MTX

---

[a] Frequent patient monitoring will prevent severe hematological abnormalities and bone marrow suppression.

Lastly, it is important to remember that the goal of the therapist is to reduce the disease burden enough to make the patient comfortable. The goal is not complete clearing of the disease. Hence, an attempt should be made to stop treatment whenever possible and after the desired therapeutic response has been achieved.

Dermatomyositis

Introduction

Dermatomyositis and polymyositis are the least common of the rheumatic/connective tissue diseases. They are primarily associated with inflammation of skeletal muscle. Patients with dermatomyositis also have an accompanying skin disease. Skeletal muscle is damaged by infiltrates of lymphocytes. Symmetry and proximal muscle weakness are characteristic, and occasionally pain is associated. Dermatomyositis and polymyositis are classified into six categories: a) primary idiopathic dermatomyositis; b) primary idiopathic polymyositis; c) polymyositis and dermatomyositis associated with malignant neoplasms; d) juvenile dermatomyositis or polymyositis; e) dermatomyositis or polymyositis associated with other rheumatic/connective tissue diseases; and f) myopathic dermatomyositis.

Disagreement exists among dermatologists and rheumatologists regarding the association of myositis and malignant neoplasms. In dermatological practice, dermatitis followed by myositis is often the presenting manifestation of disease in patients with malignancy. Additionally, a variety of retrospective studies have shown that malignancy will occur in approximately 15% of patients with myositis. Malignancies that are associated with myositis are found most often in the lungs, ovaries, breasts and gastrointestinal tract.

Primary idiopathic dermatomyositis and polymyositis can occur at any age, and are seen more often in women than men. The mean age at presentation is 50 years. The initial presentation in the two diseases is the same, except there is no skin disease evident in polymyositis. Muscle weakness begins insidiously in proximal muscle groups of the upper and lower extremities. Early on, patients complain of difficulty raising the head from the supine position or exhaustion while combing the hair. Later they experience difficulty upon arising from a chair or while climbing stairs. In dermatomyositis, striated muscle of the cricopharyngeal area is severely inflamed, resulting in difficulty initiating the swallowing reflex.

The skin lesions of dermatomyositis are fairly unique. The facial rash is often quite subtle consisting of a faint purple to red discoloration of the upper eyelids, often described as heliotropic in color. Severe disease may be associated with blister formation and erosions and scars on the upper eyelids. The lower eyelids may be edematous and quite puffy. A skin eruption may be seen over proximal muscle groups that varies from morbilliform to "lupus-like". This eruption is often associated with intense pruritus. Over the interphalangeal joints one may find one or more poly-gonal-shaped papules. These are called Gotron's papules and are a pathognomonic finding in dermatomyositis.

Childhood dermatomyositis is rarely, if ever, associated with malignancy. It is found more often in boys than girls. The gastrointestinal tract is found to be involved more often than in adult disease. Arthritis and Raynaud's phenomenon are quite frequently associated and deposition of calcium in the skin causing large, often painful, nodules occurs with considerable frequency. Many of the differences between adult and childhood disease may be accounted for by the presence of a vasculitis involving muscle groups in children.

Pathology

Pathologically the skin findings of dermatomyositis may vary from that of a mild non-specific dermatitis to the classical appearance of lupus ery-thematosus. In muscle, there is an infiltrate consisting predominantly of perivascular accumulations of lymphocytes, plasma cells, histiocytes, eosinophils, and neutrophils. There is also microscopic evidence that even as necrosis of muscle fibers is taking place, regeneration of striated muscle is occuring. Laboratory findings include increased serum levels of creatinine phosphokinase (CPK), aldolase, and transaminase (SGOT, SGPT) and an increased erythrocyte sedimentation rate. The technique of electromyography is often helpful in detecting muscle groups that are in-flamed by disease.

Etiology and pathogenesis

The autoimmune nature of dermatomyositis/polymyositis is suggested by the presence of a variety of circulating antibodies. Antibodies to nuclear antigen often give a positive antinuclear antibody test (ANA). Antibodies to Jo-1 (directed to the enzyme histidyl tRNA synthetase) occur in patients with myositis and pulmonary disease, and antibodies to n-RNP are seen in patients with myositis and other rheumatic/connective tissue diseases. Antibodies to small ribonucleoproteins Ro (SS-A) and La (SS-B) may also be observed. To date, there have been no specific antibodies found that are directed against striated muscle. Other findings that suggest autoimmunity include the presence of a polymyositis syndrome that can be produced in rats and guinea pigs immunized with skeletal muscle. A similar syndrome has been induced in laboratory animals through the transfer of sensitized lymphocytes. Lymphocytes from muscle obtained from patients with polymyositis produce a toxic lymphokine that is injurious to monolayers of human fetal muscle cells. The implication is that some form of cellular immunity and inflammation are involved in the pathogenesis of dermatomyositis and thus the efficacy of MTX in this disease.

The association of dermatomyositis polymyositis with malignant neoplasms and with other rheumatic/connective tissue disease also suggests autoimmunity.

Indications for use of methotrexate in dermatomyositis

Methotrexate is the third most commonly used agent in dermatomyositis [17]. It is favored by dermatologists, probably because of their vast experience using the drug in psoriasis.

Corticosteroids, particularly prednisone at 60–80 mg/day, have been used as the agents of choice in the treatment of dermatomyositis/polymyositis [18]. The response rate is high, yielding remission rates on the order of 90–95%. Cytotoxic agents such as MTX are indicated in that patient population with corticosteroid non-responsiveness who continue to develop destructive muscle disease. MTX is also indicated in that population of patients who require continuous moderate to high-dose prednisone as maintenance therapy. It should be pointed out that in the management of patients with dermatomyositis, patients with muscle disease and malignancy often require two to three times the normal dosage of systemic corticosteroids than patients without associated malignancy.

Cutaneous T-cell lymphoma (mycosis fungoides)

Introduction

Mycosis fungoides is a chronic malignancy that involves multifocal proliferation of T-helper cells within the skin of the host. Disease progression is manifested by the development of multiple plaques, ulcerations and tumors in sites that previously contained red scaling pruritic patches, and in the development of abnormal T-cell infiltrates in lymph nodes, liver, and spleen. Late stage disease may show abnormal T-cell infiltrates in nearly all organ systems. Intense pruritus is the hallmark of early disease.

Histologically malignant T-cell infiltrates contain large numbers of variable sized T-cells with characteristic convolutions of cell nuclei, i.e. "cerebriform nuclei" (Sézary's cells). A hematological variant (Sézary's Syndrome) in some patients may present with red, edematous skin, keratodermas of the palms and soles and large numbers of abnormal cells with cerebriform nuclei in peripheral blood (over 20% of peripheral blood white cells).

Cutaneous disease without internal organ involvement may be responsive to a variety of topical agents and physical modalities. However, cutaneous disease may become refractory to therapeutic agents and modalities directed solely toward the skin. Treatment of refractory skin disease and advanced disease is a challenge. Refractory skin disease as well as disease that has become systemic will require systemic, and/or combined topical and systemic therapy to achieve disease control.

In 1978, McDonald and Bertino reported especially good results treating mycosis fungoides with a regimen of intravenous or oral methotrexate followed by administration of leucovorin [3]. Eleven of the eleven patients achieved good to excellent clearing with minimal toxicity. Most patients were followed for a period of 24 months. This method of treatment continues to serve as the prime systemic method for treatment of patients with mycosis fungoides under our supervision. The MTX leucovorin regimen, when used regularly, remains effective for long periods and continues to show very little patient toxicity.

Over a decade and a half later, Schappell, Alper and McDonald reported on the use of MTX, 5-FU and Leucovorin for patients with advanced mycosis fungoides and Sézary's Syndrome [19]. This group tested the effectiveness of the synergy that had previously been demonstrated between MTX and 5-FU in the treatment of advanced cancerous disease. The authors' report in a group of ten patients treated from three to 78 months that the average survival for patients with tumors was 5.25 years with a mean survival of six years. Eight of the ten patients achieved at least 80% clearing, the remaining four achieved at least 60% clearing of their disease. Adverse reactions were minimal. Mucositis and leukopenia was observed in only one of the ten patients.

Polyarteritis nodosa and granulomatous vasculitis

Introduction

Polyarteritis nodosa is an inflammatory necrotizing disease that involves small and medium sized arteries in multiple organ sites [20]. Cutaneous lesions as a presenting sign in systemic disease is rare, occurring in less than 5% of patients. Late stage diseases will show cutaneous lesions in up to 50% of patients. There is a disease in which patients develop lesions of blood vessels confined only to the skin, this entity is called cutaneous polyarteritis nodosa [21].

Because polyarteritis nodosa is a multisystem disease, a variety of organs will manifest signs and symptoms. Kidney involvement is high, causing up to 50% of deaths from the disease. Gastrointestinal infarctions secondary to vasculitis is also a leading cause of death. Cardiovascular and neurological disease are associated with characteristic signs and symptoms. Lung involvement is rare.

Wegener's granulomatosis is a vasculitis associated with granulomatous inflammation in the upper and lower respiratory tract and kidneys. Inflammation in these sites produces nasal, oral, and pulmonary nodules, infiltrates and cavitary lesions in the respiratory system, and hematuria in the urinary system. Skin lesions are noted in 50% or more of patients but are generally not an initial finding.

Pathogenesis

It is postulated that the vasculitis seen in periarteritis nodosa and other vasculitides is related to an immune complex-mediated disorder [22, 23]. Other evidence suggests that immune complexes may not be the primary pathogenetic mechanism. Direct damage to blood vessels from associated inflammation of endothelial cells by platelets and platelet-derived factors and cytokines may be primary. Autoantibody to endothelial cells have been observed, as well as mast cell-basophilic cell interactions along with the production of cytokines, adhesion molecules and increased fibrinolytic activity within blood vessels [24, 25]. It appears that the use of MTX in the vasculitides reduces the inflammation so characteristic of vessels involved in these diseases. Because of the non-specific nature of the disease process in periarteritis nodosa there are no truly diagnostic serological tests available. Antineutrophilic cytoplasmic autoantibodies have been found in some vasculitides, especially Wegener's granulomatosis. Diagnosis is generally made based on the microscopic examination of tissue from multiple organ sites such as skin, nerve, and muscle combined with arteriograms.

Unlike polyarteritis nodosa, antineutrophilic cytoplasmic autoantibodies are found with some frequency in Wegener's granulomatosis [26]. These antibodies produce a cytoplasmic fluorescence pattern in most patients with Wegener's granulomatosis. Titers of antibody follow disease activity and can be used as a guide to treatment [27].

Immunomodulatory agents are indicated for use in the vasculitides as steroid-sparing agents, and in patients who have failed standard therapy.

MTX, in weekly low doses of 7.5–15 mg, has been used to supplant the use of corticosteroids [28], or in doses of 15–25 mg per week in combination with corticosteroids [29].

Miscellaneous diseases

Pemphigus vulgaris, pemphigus foliaceus and pemphigus erythematosus are a group of blistering diseases that principally affect the skin of elderly patients. Pemphigus vulgaris often involves the mucous membranes of the oral cavity, whereas such findings are rare in erythematosus and foliaceus types. Each disease appears to have an autoimmune association. Affected patients have circulating antibody, mostly IgG, directed toward cutaneous intercellular cementing substances or binding organelles resulting in the loss of cohesion between epidermal cells. These immune globulins, which appear to be pathogenic, may be detected by direct and indirect immuno-fluorescent methods. Antibody titers often correlate closely with disease activity. Patients with severe, rapidly progressive disease, and those who are non-responsive to high doses of corticosteroids are considered candidates for treatment with one or more immunosuppresive agents [30]. In 1969, Lever and others proposed the use of MTX for patients with pemphigus vulgaris [4]. This period was followed by a decade of intense popularity in which MTX was almost routinely used to treat pemphigus. However, in recent years, the use of other more potent immunosuppresive agents have supplanted the use of MTX in pemphigus [31].

Pityriasis rubra pilaris (PRP) is an uncommon papulo-squamous disorder of the skin with an unknown etiology. In typical patients the disease begins as clusters of red plaques and follicular papules that ultimately coalesce, progressing to generalized erythroderma over variable time periods. Histologically one sees a very sparse dermal perivascular infiltrate of lymphocytes and histiocytes, ortho-and parakeratosis, hypergranulosis, thick suprapapillary plates, broad rete ridges and narrow dermal papillae. Although the cause is unknown, the fundamental abnormality appears to be epidermal hyperproliferation [32].

MTX has been used widely to treat PRP although clinical response rates have not been as consistent as seen in psoriasis. Current treatment dosage schedules are comparable to those used in psoriasis.

Sarcoidosis is a disease with protean manifestations. It may occur primarily in the skin, or may involve the skin and multiple organ systems. It, like secondary and tertiary syphilis may mimic a variety of cutaneous diseases such as lupus erythematosus, psoriasis, syphilis, and tuberculosis. The disease is often seen in patients of Scandinavian and African-American heritage. It is quite common in the southeastern part of the United States. Cutaneous lesions frequently occur as papules around the eyes and the oral cavity. They may also occur at sites of trauma. Nodular lesions scattered over the trunk of an affected patient are often of the granulomatous type. Pulmonary hilar adenopathy and infiltrates may be observed. Histopathologically the disease is characterized by infiltrates of inflammatory cells, mostly T-cells and histiocytes. Fibrosis is often seen in older cutaneous and systemic lesions. Collections of inflammatory and histocytic cells often form micro-nodules. Like other diseases of an inflammatory nature, sarcoidosis responds to treatment with corticosteroids. Hence, these agents have become the drugs of choice for the treatment of cutaneous and systemic disease. Cytotoxic drugs have been used to aid in the control of disease refractory to corticosteroids and as steroid – sparing agents. Veien and Brodthagen have reported on the use of MTX in sarcoidosis [33]. In our experience, although not the cytotoxic agent of choice, MTX is an effective drug in a program of combined agents designed to control the external and internal manifestations of sarcoidosis.

Summary

During the past two-to-three decades, MTX has been found to be a very useful, relatively safe and effective agent in the management of patients with a variety of skin diseases. Most of these diseases are characterized by altered immunity, cellular hyperplasia and inflammation. Among dermatologists MTX is the most widely used agent of its type, its use being exceeded only by its use in the treatment of neoplastic diseases.

References

1 Rees RB, Bennett JH, Bostick WL (1955) Aminopterin for psoriasis. Arch Dermat 72: 133–143
2 McDonald CJ, Bertino JR. (1969) Parenteral methotrexate in psoriasis. Arch Dermat 100: 655–668
3 McDonald CJ, Bertino JR. (1978) Treatment of mycosis fungoides lymphoma: effectiveness of infusions of methotrexate followed by oral citrovorum factor leucovorin. Cancer Treatment Reports 62 (7): 1009–1014
4 Lever WF, Goldberg HS (1969) Treatment of pemphigus vulgaris with methotrexate. Arch Dermat 100: 70–78
5 Jorizzo JL, White WL, Wise CM (1991) Low-dose weekly methotrexate for unusual neutrophilic vascular reactions: cutaneous polyarteritis and Behcet's disease. J Am Acad Dermat 24: 973–978
6 Knowles WR, Chernasky ME (1970) Pityriasis rubra pilaris, prolonged treatment with methotrexate. Arch Dermat 102: 603–612
7 Rea JN, Newhouse ML, Halil T (1976) Skin disease in Lambeth: a community study of prevalence and use of medical care. Br J Prev Soc Med 30: 107–114

8 Weinstein GD, McCullough JL (1991) Cell proliferation kinetics. In: HH Jr Roenigk, HI Maibach (eds): *Psoriasis*. 2nd ed. Marcel Dekker, New York, 327–342

9 Cooper KD (1990) Psoriasis: leucocytes and cytokines. *Dermat Clin* 8: 737–745

10 Braverman IM (1985) Microcirculation. In: HH Jr Roenigk, HI Maibach (eds): *Psoriasis*. Marcel Dekker, New York, 287–298

11 el-Sherif AI, Krupinski P, Majewski S, Jablonska S (1994) Leucocyte-extracellular matrix interactions in psoriasis. *Int J Dermat* 33: 371–373

12 Schlaak JF, Buslau M, Jochum W, Hermann E, Girndt M (1994) T-cells in psoriasis vulgaris belong to the TH 1 subset. *J Invest Dermat* 102: 145–159

13 Nickoloff BJ (1991) The cytokine network in psoriasis. *Arch Dermat* 127: 871–884

14 Krueger JG, Krane JF, Carter DM, Gottlieb AB (1990) Role of growth factors, cytokines and their receptors in the pathogenesis of psoriasis. *J Invest Dermat* 94 (Suppl): 135S–140S

15 Weinstein GD, Krueger JG (1993) An overview of psoriasis. In: GD Weinstein, AB Gottlieb (eds): *Therapy of moderate to severe psoriasis*. National Psoriasis Foundation, Portland, OR 1–23

16 Zachariae H, Sogaard H (1987) Methotrexate-induced liver cirrhosis: a follow up. *Dermatologica* 175: 178–182

17 Miller LC, Sisson BA, Tucker BA (1992) Methotrexate treatment of recalcitrant childhood dermatomyositis. *Arthr Rheum* 35: 1143–1149

18 Boyd AS, Nelder KH (1994) Therapeutic options in dermatomyositis/polymyositis. *Int J Dermat* 33: 240–250

19 Schappell DL, Alper JC, McDonald CJ (1995) Treatment of advanced mycosis fungoides and Sézary syndrome with continuous infusions of methotrexate followed by fluorouracil and leucovorin rescue. *Arch Dermat* 131 (3): 307–313

20 Jennett CJ, Milling DM, Falk RJ (1994) Vasculitis affecting the skin. *Arch Dermat* 130: 899–906

21 Diaz-Perez JL, Winkelmann RK (1974) Cutaneous periarteritis nodosa. *Arch Dermat* 110: 407–414

22 Kammer GM, Soter NA, Schur PH (1980) Circulating immune complexes in patients with necrotizing vasculitis. *Clin Immunol Immunopathol* 15: 658–670

23 Braverman IM, Yen A (1975) Demonstration of immune complexes in spontaneous and histamine-induced lesions and in normal skin of patients with leukocytoclastic angiitis. *J Invest Dermat* 64: 105–112

24 Kallenberg CGM (1993) Autoantibodies in vasculitis: current perspectives. *Clin Exp Rheum* 11: 355–360

25 Jordan JM, Allen NB, Pizo SV (1987) Defective release of tissue plasminogen activator in systemic and cutaneous vasculitis. *Am J Med* 82: 397–400

26 van der Woude TJ, Rasmussen N, Lobatto S (1985) Autoantibodies against neutrophils and monycytes: tool for diagnosis and marker of disease activity in Wegener's granulomatosis. *Lancet* 1: 425–429

27 Cohen TJW, Huitema MG, Hené RJ (1990) Prevention of relapses in Wegener's granulomatosis by treatment based on antineutrophil cytoplasmic antibody titre. *Lancet* 336: 709–711

28 Jorizzo JL, White WL, Wise CM (1991) Low-dose weekly methotrexate for unusual neutrophilic vascular reactions: cutaneous polyarteritis and Behcet's disease. *J Am Acad Dermat* 24: 973–978

29 Hoffman GS, Leavitt RY, Kerr GS, Fauci AS (1992) The treatment of Wegener's granulomatosis with glucocorticoids and methotrexate. *Arthr Rheum* 35: 1322–1329

30 Mobini N, Ahmed AR (1997) Bullous diseases: pathogenesis and treatment. In: McDonald CJ (ed): *Immunomodulatory and cytotoxic agents in dermatology*. Marcel Dekker, New York, 169–190

31 Bystryn JC (1985) Adjuvant therapy of pemphigus. *Arch Dermat* 120: 941–951

32 Griffiths WA, Pieris S (1982) Pityriasis rubra pilaris – an autoradiographic study. *Br J Dermat* 107 (6): 665–667

33 Veien NK, Brodthagen H (1977) Cutaneous sarcoidosis treated with methotrexate. *Br J Dermat* 97: 213–216

Methotrexate
ed. by B. N. Cronstein und J. R. Bertino
© 2000 Birkhäuser Verlag Basel/Switzerland

The use of methotrexate in gynecological practice

Ana Monteagudo and Ilan E. Timor-Tritsch

Department of Obstetrics and Gynecology, New York University Medical Center, 550 First Avenue Rm 9N26, New York, NY 10023, USA

Introduction

In gynecological practice the use of methotrexate was confined to the treatment of malignancies until 1982 when the first report of the use of methotrexate to treat an interstitial pregnancy was reported [1]. Since that time the use of methotrexate to treat tubal, cervical, and interstitial pregnancies has become widely accepted and practiced in many centers around the world. In addition, methotrexate has been used to treat pregnancies implanted within a uterine scar and in patients with placenta accreta. However, in this chapter we will limit the discussion to the use of methotrexate in the treatment of ectopic pregnancies.

The revolution that has occurred in assisted reproductive technologies has in turn resulted in an explosion in the number, types and varieties of ectopic pregnancies that are being diagnosed. Therefore, the outpatient use of methotrexate to treat ectopic pregnancies has increased dramatically over the last ten years. There are many reasons for the increased use of non-surgical treatments: decreased operative morbidity, improved fertility and, lastly, decreased surgical costs. Of course, not everyone is supportive of non-surgical treatments of ectopic pregnancies. Those who are frankly opposed to this treatment give one or more of the following reasons: 1) the potential toxicity of methotrexate; 2) the potential long-term reproductive effects of the drug; 3) the need for patient follow-up and monitoring; 4) the risk of treatment failure; 5) the treatment-associated pain; 6) the lack of a cost outcome analysis and 7) the uncertain diagnostic reliability in the absence of laparoscopy [2]. There are also other, mainly non-medical reasons for not adopting it.

At present there is no single protocol accepted and practiced by all institutions with regard to the administration of methotrexate. In some institutions the medication has been injected directly into the ectopic pregnancy under laparoscopic or transvaginal sonographic guidance while in other institutions the medication is given intramuscularly, intravenously or orally. Some protocols call for relatively high doses of methotrexate, while in others the doses are relatively low.

This chapter will review the use of methotrexate in ectopic pregnancies and try to familiarize the reader with the most widely used protocols and indications for the medical treatment of ectopic pregnancies.

Tubal ectopic pregnancies

In the United States tubal ectopic pregnancies account for approximately 2% of all pregnancies [3]. This type of pregnancy is associated with a significant amount of morbidity and even mortality for the mother, although maternal mortality rates have fallen sharply in the United States over the last 30 years from approximately 63 per 10,000 in 1970 to 30 per 10,000 in 1987 [4]. During the first trimester of pregnancy ectopic pregnancy is the leading cause of maternal deaths and accounts for 9–13% of all pregnancy related deaths [5]. Risk factors for ectopic pregnancies include pelvic inflammatory disease, tubal surgery, *in utero* exposure to diethylstilbestrol, sexually transmitted diseases, pharmacological treatment of infertility, assisted reproductive technologies such as *in vitro* fertilization and gamete intrafallopian transfer, endometriosis, and impaired ciliary function from the use of intrauterine contraceptives [4, 6, 7].

Treatment for tubal ectopic pregnancies has evolved over the last century from the invasive laparotomy with salpingectomy to the more conservative treatment of laparoscopic salpingectomy, or salpingostomy. The problem with these more conservative surgical treatments is the risk of subsequent ectopic pregnancies that may occur in approximately 5% [8] to 10% of patients [9, 10] and that of persistent ectopic pregnancies that may occur in as few as 3% [11] and as many as 20% of the cases [12]. In these patients with persistent ectopic pregnancies further medical treatment with methotrexate is indicated. In a review published in 1992 five percent of the patients did not respond to methotrexate and ended up having surgery [13].

The medical treatment of ectopic pregnancies began in 1982 when Tanaka [1] and his colleagues first reported the successful treatment of an interstitial pregnancy using intramuscular (IM) methotrexate. During the next few years many case reports of successful cases of ectopic pregnancies treated with methotrexate were published.

Medical or non-surgical treatment of ectopic pregnancy has become a reality due to the fact that, at present, the reliable diagnosis of ectopic pregnancy can be made effectively without the use of laparoscopy, culdocentesis or dilatation and curettage (D & C). The reliable diagnosis of ectopic pregnancy became possible with the introduction of two laboratory tests, namely transvaginal sonography [14, 15] and the quantitative serum level of human chorionic gonadotropin (hCG) [16–18]. In addition to these two tests, serum progesterone concentration has also been used because in cases of ectopic pregnancy the level is lower (< 15 ng/mL) than in viable intrauterine pregnancies (≥ 15 ng/mL) [19, 20].

The first series of patients treated by methotrexate were those of Miyazaki in 1983 [21] and subsequently Ory et al. in 1986 [22]. Miyazaki [21] reported on the non-surgical treatment of nine patients with tubal ectopic pregnancy using methotrexate (MTX). Total doses of 60–300 mg provided complete remission in eight cases; the other underwent salpingectomy due to the progression of abortion. In the cases with hCG titer below 1,000 IU/l the dose of MTX used was 60–105 mg, however, in those cases with hCG over 4,000 IU/l the dose of MTX used was 75–300 mg. Patency of fallopian tubes after the regimen was confirmed in five out of six cases with hystero-salpingography. Subsequently, Ory and colleagues [22] reported on six patients with distal ampullary ectopic pregnancies that were treated with four doses of intravenous methotrexate (1.0 mg/kg) followed by four doses of leucovorin (0.1 mg/kg, intramuscularly). The diagnosis of ectopic pregnancy was established in all cases by laparoscopy following sonography and radioimmunoassay for serum β-hCG (beta subunit of human chorionic gonadotropin). Five of the six patients experienced resolution of their ectopic pregnancy without additional surgical treatment. One patient underwent salpingectomy following treatment. Other types of morbidity encountered included three patients with mild stomatitis or gastritis, and two patients had transient elevations of serum transaminase levels. Two patients had protracted courses and received blood transfusions. The most abrupt response and most uncomplicated courses were experienced in the three subjects with initial human chorionic gonadotropin levels below 1000 mIU/ml. These authors concluded that methotrexate may be an effective alternative for the treatment of early ectopic pregnancy.

Stovall and his colleagues were the first group to report on the use of "single dose" of methotrexate to treat ectopic pregnancies [2, 23–25]. However, this description of the clinical practice is not exactly correct since a significant number of patients in most series reported required a second dose of methotrexate to achieve resolution. Initially, Stovall reported on the treatment of 30 patients with unruptured ectopic pregnancy, measuring 3.5 cm or less, using a single dose of intramuscular methotrexate (50 mg/ m^2) without leucovorin rescue. Pre-treatment hCG titers ranged from 130–16,700 mIU/mL (mean 4558). Pre-treatment transvaginal sonography visualized the ectopic pregnancy in 28 of 30 patients (93.3%) and revealed cardiac activity in six patients. Patients were monitored with hCG titers three times per week for the first week, and then weekly until the hCG was less than 15 mIU/mL. A complete blood count and liver enzymes were obtained before treatment and on day seven. All patients had a continued rise in hCG titer for at least three days after methotrexate injection, although all levels began to decline by day seven. No patient required a second dose of methotrexate and no patient experienced any side effects. Twenty-nine of the 30 patients (96.7%) were successfully treated [23].

Subsequently, in 1993 Stovall et al. [25] published his expanded clinical trial using a single-dose of 50 mg/m^2 intramuscular methotrexate without leucovorin factor rescue for the treatment of unruptured ectopic pregnancies. This study involved a prospective cohort of 120 women with an ectopic pregnancy ≤3.5 cm in size. Inclusion criteria were: 1) the patients had to be hemodynamically stable; 2) if performed, the hCG titer increased after a curettage; 3) transvaginal sonography demonstrated an unruptured ectopic pregnancy of ≤ 3.5 cm in size; 4) the patients desired future fertility and 5) had signed informed consent. The exclusion criteria were: 1) the patients had declining hCG titers after curettage; 2) transvaginal sonography demonstrated an ectopic pregnancy of > 3.5 cm in size; 3) the patients were hemodynamically unstable; 4) they did not desired future fertility and 5) had evidence of hepatic dysfunction, blood dyscrasia, thrombocytopenia or renal disease. Follow-up for the patients with ≥ 15% decline in hCG titers between days four and seven were followed-up weekly until the hCG titer was ≤ 12 mIU/ml. If there was a decline of < 15% or a rise in the hCG level or the hCG level plateaued, a second intramuscular dose of methotrexate (50 mg/m^2) was given on day seven. The results were as follows: the mean hCG titer before treatment initiation was 3950 ± 1193 mIU/ml. Transvaginal ultrasonography demonstrated cardiac activity in 14 (11.7%) patients, with an ectopic mass visualized in 113 (94.2%). The mean time to resolution in the 113 (94.2%) subjects successfully treated was 35.5 ± 11.8 days. Four (3.3%) patients required a second methotrexate dose on day seven. No biochemical or clinical side effects occurred. Posttreatment hysterosalpingograms demonstrated tubal patency on the ipsilateral side in 51 of the 62 (82.3%) patients. Of those attempting pregnancy, 79.6% were pregnant, 87.2% intrauterine and 12.8% ectopic. The mean time to achieve pregnancy was 3.2 ± 1.1 months. The conclusion of this paper was that this regimen of methotrexate requires minimal laboratory follow-up and eliminates leukovorin recovery, making it the regimen of choice for medical treatment of unruptured ectopic pregnancy.

Recently, Lipscomb et al. [26] published the largest series, comprising of 315 patients (this included the patients previously reported by Stovall), of unruptured ectopic pregnancies treated with a single dose of methotrexate (50 mg/m^2). Overall, 287 patients were successfully treated with methotrexate for a success rate of 90.1%. Six patients electively withdrew and requested surgery within one week of starting therapy. Excluding the patients who withdrew, the overall success rate was 92.9%. Ten patients with an ectopic pregnancy > 3.5 cm but ≤ 4 cm in size were treated with a 90% success rate. Forty-four patients with positive ectopic cardiac activity were treated with an 87.5% success rate. They concluded that single-dose intramuscular methotrexate for treatment of ectopic pregnancy is associated with an excellent overall success rate.

Parker et al. [27] performed a systematic review of all available studies and case reports of intramuscular methotrexate to examine the therapeutic efficacy, side-effects and complication rates of this new treatment approach. The pooled data show a successful resolution rate of 71% (95% confidence interval 58% to 81%) after a single dose of intramuscular methotrexate and 84% (95% confidence interval 77% to 90%) after one or two doses. Side-effects were experienced by 24% (95% confidence interval 9% to 47%) of patients and 10% (95% confidence interval 7% to 14%)

had a ruptured ectopic pregnancy. The pooled data show that single-dose intramuscular methotrexate is associated with a high failure rate. Follow-up is prolonged and there is a significant incidence of minor side-effects. Serious complications and side-effects have occurred. Complications include worsening pain and tubal rupture. Exacerbation of pain was found in 40% of patients after a single dose of methotrexate and tubal rupture in up to 10% of the pooled cases. Tubal rupture was unrelated to the ultra-sound size of the ectopic pregnancy and may occur with declining hCG levels. They concluded from the pooled data that the use of intramuscular methotrexate should be confined to clinical trials until more evidence is obtained to support its more widespread use.

The first report of a local injection of methotrexate under transvaginal sonographic guidance was by Feichtinger and Kemeter in 1987. They reported on the successful treatment of an ampullary ectopic pregnancy of a patient that had undergone *in vitro* fertilization (IVF) using 10 ml of methotrexate directly into the ectopic pregnancy [28]. The reported success rates of local injection under ultrasound guidance ranges from 70% to 95% [29–32].

Merz et al. [33] treated 30 patients locally with methotrexate under sono-graphic guidance. Local methotrexate therapy was successful in 25 patients (83.3%). Eighteen of these patients had received a single methotrexate instillation with a total dose of 10 mg, seven patients had received a second instillation with 10 mg because of plateau hCG levels after the first in-stillation. In five patients methotrexate therapy was unsuccessful. Surgical intervention was necessary within 4 h to 15 days after methotrexate treat-ment, due to severe tubal bleeding $(n = 1)$ or the development of an in-creasing peritubal hematoma $(n = 4)$. Patients with an outer trophoblast diameter ≤ 1.5 cm could be treated successfully in all cases (25/25). In patients with hCG values $> 5,000$ mIU/ml the success rate was 70% (7/10) and in patients with a demonstration of cardiac activity of the embryo 63% (5/8). The decline in hCG to values below 10 mIU/ml ranged between seven and 75 days (mean 28 days). The hysterosalpingography performed 4–6 months after methotrexate therapy showed tubal patency on both sides in 85.7% of the patients examined. In the meantime four of these patients gave birth to healthy children.

Mesogitis et al. [34] treated 26 tubal pregnancies with local methotrexate injection. A single dose of 10–12.5 mg of methotrexate was percutaneous-ly injected into the gestational sac under abdominal sonographic control. Complete resolution was obtained in all patients. Four of them required a second percutaneous administration four days after the first one. No systemic side effects were observed. Local administration of methotrexate under abdominal sonographic control seems to be an effective alternative for the treatment of ectopic pregnancy. The main potential advantages of the method are (1) a greater antitrophoblastic effect; (2) a shorter treatment period; (3) reduced dosage, and (4) absence of side effects.

Pisarska et al. in 1998 [35] reviewed the literature dealing with management of ectopic pregnancies. Medical management of ectopic pregnancy included variable-dose methotrexate, a single dose of methotrexate or local injection of methotrexate. She identified 12 studies (one randomized controlled trial, one cohort study, and ten case series) in which a variable-dose methotrexate was used to treat tubal ectopic pregnancies (Tabs. 1, 2). Of the total 338 cases identified, 93% were successfully treated with variable doses of methotrexate. The rates of tubal patency and subsequent fertility were similar to those with conservative surgical management, though the rate of subsequent ectopic pregnancy was lower. She reviewed seven studies of single-dose methotrexate (one cohort, and six case-control studies). Combining these studies yielded 393 patients with a mean success rate of 87%

Table 1. Medical treatment with methotrexate[a]

Indication
  Diameter ≤ 4 cm
  β-hcg rising at 48 h
  Normal blood count, platelets and liver enzymes.

Procedure
  Variable dose
  Methotrexate 1 mg/kg intramuscularly, alternate days (days 1, 3, 5, 7)
  Leucovorin 0.1 mg/kg intramuscularly, alternate days (2, 4, 6, 8)
  Continue until β-hcg falls $\geq 15\%$ in 48 h or four doses methotrexate given

  Single dose
  Methotrexate 50 mg/m^2 intramuscularly
  Repeat dose if β-hcg on day 7 $\geq$ day 4

Follow-up
  Weekly β-hcg until <5 IU/L
  No sexual intercourse, pelvic examinations, or ultrasonography until resolved.
  Repeat course for persistent ectopic pregnancy.

[a] Modified after [35].

Table 2. Outcome of treatment for ectopic pregnancy[a]

Method	Studies	Patients	Successful	Tubal patency	Subsequent fertility	
					IUP	Ectopic
Variable dose methotrexate	12	338	314 (93%)	136/182 (75%)	55/95 (58%)	7/95 (7%)
Single-dose methotrexate	7	393	340 (87%)	61/75 (61%)	39/64 (61%)	5/64 (8%)
Direct-injection methotrexate	21	660	502 (76%)	130/162 (80%)	87/152 (57%)	9/152 (6%)

[a] Modified after [35].

(patients not requiring surgical intervention), however, 8% of the patients required a second dose of methotrexate. She included in her paper 21 studies with a total of 660 patients where the rates of successful treatment were lower than for systemic methotrexate. In my experience the only indication for *injecting* methotrexate into a tubal ectopic pregnancy, is if there is a live tubal ectopic pregnancy otherwise systemic methotrexate should be considered the route of choice.

Cervical and cornual ectopic pregnancies

Cervical and cornual ectopic pregnancies, although not as common as tubal pregnancies, can both result in significant morbidity and mortality.

Cervical pregnancies

Among the ectopic pregnancies cervical pregnancy is the most dreaded by obstetricians. This is due to the fact that a life threatening hemorrhage can occur. Cervical pregnancy is a rare event with a reported incidence of 1/1000 to 1/18,000 [36].They comprise approximately 0.15% of all ectopic pregnancies. However, the true incidence of cervical pregnancies is probably unknown due to under-reporting. The etiology of cervical pregnancy has not been clearly elucidated. However, a history of factors such as dilatation and curettage, Cesarean section, intrauterine device and *in vitro* fertilization is frequently encountered [37–43]. Using transvaginal sonography the diagnosis of a viable cervical pregnancy can be made when the following sonographic criteria are met: 1) the placenta and the entire chorionic sac containing a live fetus is below the internal os. The level of the internal os is considered to be at the level of the insertion of the uterine arteries; 2) the uterine cavity is empty; and 3) the cervical canal is significantly dilated and barrel shaped [39].

Over the last ten years, with the increased use and availability of ultrasound, the diagnosis of cervical pregnancy has been made at earlier gestational ages and in many instances when the patient is totally asymptomatic and stable. Detection of cervical pregnancy in these asymptomatic or minimally symptomatic patients has resulted in an increase in therapeutic options and enabled the use of more conservative surgical approaches that aim to preserve the uterus and the patient's reproductive potential. Systemic administration of methotrexate as well as local injection into the cervical pregnancy have been described. However, experience with these treatment modalities is relatively sparse and there is no general consensus about the most effective treatment for cervical pregnancy. This is due to the fact that, unlike tubal ectopic, this is a rare problem and most of the literature on the subject consists of case reports in which methotrexate was successfully used.

Table 3. The results of non-surgical treatment of early cervical pregnancy[a]

Treatment	N	Gestation mean (weeks)	Gestation range (weeks)	Success rate %	Hemorrhage rate %	Hysterectomy rate %
Systemic methotrexate	24	7.5	5–12	19/24 (79)	3/24 (13)	1/24 (4)
Local injection of methotrexate or potassium chloride	16	7.3	5–12	13/16 (81)	1/16 (6)	0
Other systemic therapy	3	7.3	6–10	3/3 (100)	0	0
Total	43	7.4	5–12	35/43 (81)	4/43 (9)	1/43 (2)

[a] From [44].

The use of systemic methotrexate in cases of cervical ectopic pregnancy has been largely for the non-viable (absence of cardiac activity or in cases of an empty gestational sac) cervical pregnancies. The regime of methotrexate, either a variable-dose or single dose, has been the same as that used for tubal ectopic pregnancies (Tab. 1) and, similar to the tubal ectopic pregnancy, direct injection into the cervical pregnancy has been limited to those in which fetal cardiac activity is seen.

Jurkovic et al. [44] reviewed the literature in this area and reported that among the patients who were given systemic chemotherapy, the treatment failed in 5/11 (45%) patients with viable cervical pregnancies. In contrast, all 16 patients with a non-viable cervical pregnancy were treated successfully (Tab. 3).

Cornual or isthmic ectopic pregnancies

Cornual ectopic pregnancies account for 2–4% of ectopic pregnancies. This type of ectopic pregnancy, if left alone, progresses further than the tubal ectopic or cervical pregnancies. A live cornual pregnancy of 12–16 weeks is not unusual. The myometrium surrounding the cornual gestation thins as the pregnancy progresses and eventually it ruptures. Rupture of a cornual ectopic pregnancy may result in severe hemorrhage due to the abundant blood supply to this area. Cornual ectopic pregnancies, like tubal ectopic pregnancies, have been treated surgically in the past either by local excision of the cornual area of the uterus or by hysterectomy. However, patients undergoing cornual resection may be at risk of uterine rupture in subsequent pregnancies. Ultrasound, especially transvaginal sonography, allows an early diagnosis before the pregnancy has progressed into the second trimester and enables "conservative medical management". By this we mean injection of live cornual pregnancies with methotrexate or, similar to the medical treatment of cervical pregnancies, non-viable cornual ectopic pregnancies may be treated with systemic methotrexate. The doses used are similar to those for the treatment of tubal ectopic pregnancies (Tab. 1). However, live cornual ectopic pregnancies, if treated with systemic methotrexate, have a higher failure rate. Similar to the live cervical ectopic pregnancies, this type of cornual ectopic pregnancy should be treated with local injection of methotrexate [45].

Benifla et al. [46] treated fifteen patients with clear evidence of an unruptured interstitial pregnancy by injection of methotrexate or potassium chloride (KCl) without surgery. The diagnosis was established either by sonography and laparoscopic confirmation in eight cases or by only transvaginal ultrasound in seven cases. Four different protocols of methotrexate administration were used in this series: 1) 15 mg i.m. methotrexate daily for five days was used; 2) 1 mg/kg body weight i.m. of methotrexate daily for four days; 3) 1 mg/kg body weight intratubal injection associated with 1 mg/kg body weight methotrexate i.m. daily for three days; and 4) 1 mg/kg body weight given intratubally. Success was defined as declining serum hCG to undetectable levels, and that no further surgical management was required. Outcome of subsequent fertility was also evaluated. The results showed that complete resolution was obtained in 13 (86.6%) out of 15 interstitial pregnancies. Two out of 15 patients, with failure of medical treatment, required a secondary surgery. No severe side effects of the medical treatment were observed. Follow-up hysterosalpingography was performed in 12 patients and showed 91.7% tubal patency on the side of the interstitial pregnancy. Amongst the other 12 patients in this series, nine became pregnant within one year: eight pregnancies reached term, and one resulted in an induced abortion. Among the last three patients, two had no desire to conceive. They concluded that an unruptured interstitial pregnancy can be managed with local methotrexate administration of 1 mg/kg body weight under transvaginal ultrasound guidance or under laparoscopic procedure. This puncture approach is particularly attractive in patients where the only alternative to therapy is laparotomy with cornual resection.

Heterotopic pregnancies

Over the last several years we have dealt with several cases of heterotopic pregnancies, namely an ectopic pregnancy co-existing with an intrauterine pregnancy. In these cases, for obvious reasons, the use of methotrexate locally or systemically is contraindicated therefore we have advocated treating the ectopic pregnancy with injection of potasium chloride [15, 43]. In two cases of heterotopic pregnancies (intrauterine with a cervical ectopic) we reported that the cervical pregnancy was injected with potassium chloride (2 meq/ml) using a transvaginal guided puncture procedure. Both pregnancies resulted in live born babies delivered by cesarean section at 34 and 31 weeks. In Benifla's [46] series three out of 15 cases of cornual ectopic pregnancies had a heterotopic pregnancy that were treated by transvaginal ultrasound-guided injection of potasium chloride. The outcome of the intra-uterine pregnancy of the three patients who had heterotopic gestation was: two miscarriages and one delivery at term. Baker et al. [47] terminated an interstitial pregnancy using one milliliter of 20% potasium chloride mixed with 12.5 mg of methotrexate. The interstitial pregnancy resolved, and a healthy term infant was delivered.

Conclusion

Methotrexate used systemically or locally provides another option for patients with ectopic pregnancies. This is especially important in patients with cervical or cornual ectopics which, if treated surgically, may result in a tremendous amount of blood loss or may impact on future fertility.

References

1 Tanaka T, Hayashi H, Kutsuzawa T, Fujimoto S, Ichinoe K (1982) Treatment of interstitial ectopic pregnancy with methotrexate: report of a successful case. *Fertil Steril* 37: 851–852

2 Stovall TG (1995) Medical management should be routinely used as primary therapy for ectopic pregnancy. *Clin Obstet Gynecol* 38: 346–352

3 Ectopic pregnancy – United States, 1990–1992 (1995) *Morb Mortal Wkly Rep* 44: 46–48

4 Minnick-Smith K, Cook F (1997) Current treatment options for ectopic pregnancy. *Am J Matern Child Nurs* 22: 21–25

5 Goldner TE, Lawson HW, Xia Z, Atrash HK (1993) Surveillance for ectopic pregnancy – United States, 1970–1989. *Mor Mortal Wkly Rep CDC Surveill Summ* 42: 73–85

6 Zorn JR, Risquez F, Cedard L (1992) Ectopic pregnancy. *Curr Opin Obstet Gynecol* 4: 238–245

7 Cowan BD (1993) Ectopic pregnancy. *Curr Opin Obstet Gynecol* 5: 328–332

8 Vermesh M, Presser SC (1992) Reproductive outcome after linear salpingostomy for ectopic gestation: a prospective 3-year follow-up. *Fertil Steril* 57: 682–684

9 Lundorff P, Thorburn J, Hahlin M, Kallfelt B, Lindblom B (1991) Laparoscopic surgery in ectopic pregnancy. A randomized trial vs. laparotomy. *Acta Obstet Gynecol Scand* 70: 343–348

10 Lundorff P, Thorburn J, Lindblom B (1992) Fertility outcome after conservative surgical treatment of ectopic pregnancy evaluated in a randomized trial. *Fertil Steril* 57: 998–1002

11 Vermesh M, Silva PD, Rosen GF, Stein AL, Fossum GT, Sauer MV (1989) Management of unruptured ectopic gestation by linear salpingostomy: a prospective, randomized clinical trial of laparoscopy vs. laparotomy. *Obstet Gynecol* 73: 400–404

12 Henderson SR (1989) Ectopic tubal pregnancy treated by operative laparoscopy. *Am J Obstet Gynecol* 160: 1462–1466; discussion 1466–1469

13 Kooi S, Kock HC (1992) A review of the literature on nonsurgical treatment in tubal pregnancies. *Obstet Gynecol Surv* 47: 739–749

14 Timor-Tritsch IE, Yeh MN, Peisner DB, Lesser KB, Slavik TA (1989) The use of transvaginal ultrasonography in the diagnosis of ectopic pregnancy. *Am J Obstet Gynecol* 161: 157–161

15 Timor-Tritsch IE (1998) Is it safe to use methotrexate for selective injection in heterotopic pregnancy? *Am J Obstet Gynecol* 178: 193–194

16 Romero R, Kadar N, Jeanty P, Copel JA, Chervenak FA, DeCherney A, Hobbins JC (1985) Diagnosis of ectopic pregnancy: value of the discriminatory human chorionic gonadotropin zone. *Obstet Gynecol* 66: 357–360

17 Romero R, Kadar N, Copel JA, Jeanty P, DeCherney AH, Hobbins JC (1986) The value of serial human chorionic gonadotropin testing as a diagnostic tool in ectopic pregnancy. *Am J Obstet Gynecol* 155: 392–394

18 Kadar N, DeVore G, Romero R (1981) Discriminatory hCG zone: its use in the sonographic evaluation for ectopic pregnancy. *Obstet Gynecol* 58: 156–161

19 Matthews CP, Coulson PB, Wild RA (1986) Serum progesterone levels as an aid in the diagnosis of ectopic pregnancy. *Obstet Gynecol* 68: 390–394

20 Yeko TR, Gorrill MJ, Hughes LH, Rodi IA, Buster JE, Sauer MV (1987) Timely diagnosis of early ectopic pregnancy using a single blood progesterone measurement. *Fertil Steril* 48: 1048–1050

21 Miyazaki Y (1983) Non-surgical therapy of ectopic pregnancy. *Hokkaido Igaku Zasshi* 58: 132–143

22 Ory SJ, Villanueva AL, Sand PK, Tamura RK (1986) Conservative treatment of ectopic pregnancy with methotrexate. *Am J Obstet Gynecol* 154: 1299–1306

23 Stovall TG, Ling FW, Gray LA (1991) Single-dose methotrexate for treatment of ectopic pregnancy. *Obstet Gynecol* 77: 754–757

24 Stovall TG, Ling FW, Gray LA, Carson SA, Buster JE (1991) Methotrexate treatment of unruptured ectopic pregnancy: a report of 100 cases. *Obstet Gynecol* 77: 749–753

25 Stovall TG, Ling FW (1993) Single-dose methotrexate: an expanded clinical trial. *Am J Obstet Gynecol* 168: 1759–1762; discussion 1762–1765

26 Lipscomb GH, Bran D, McCord ML, Portera JC, Ling FW (1998) Analysis of three hundred fifteen ectopic pregnancies treated with single-dose methotrexate. *Am J Obstet Gynecol* 178: 1354–1358

27 Parker J, Bisits A, Proietto AM (1998) A systematic review of single-dose intramuscular methotrexate for the treatment of ectopic pregnancy. *Aust N Z J Obstet Gynaecol* 38: 145–150

28 Feichtinger W, Kemeter P (1987) Conservative treatment of ectopic pregnancy by trans-vaginal aspiration under sonographic control and methotrexate injection. *Lancet* 1: 381–382

29 Fernandez H, Benifla JL, Lelaidier C, Baton C, Frydman R (1993) Methotrexate treatment of ectopic pregnancy: 100 cases treated by primary transvaginal injection under sono-graphic control. *Fertil Steril* 59: 773–777

30 Fernandez H, Pauthier S, Doumerc S, Lelaidier C, Olivennes F, Ville Y, Frydman R (1995) Ultrasound-guided injection of methotrexate vs. laparoscopic salpingotomy in ectopic pregnancy. *Fertil Steril* 63: 25–29

31 Tulandi T, Atri M, Bret P, Falcone T, Khalife S (1992) Transvaginal intratubal methotrexate treatment of ectopic pregnancy. *Fertil Steril* 58: 98–100

32 Menard A, Crequat J, Mandelbrot L, Hauuy JP, Madelenat P (1990) Treatment of unruptured tubal pregnancy by local injection of methotrexate under transvaginal sonographic control. *Fertil Steril* 54: 47–50

33 Merz E, Bahlmann F, Weber G, Macchiella D, Kruczynski D, Pollau K, Knapstein PG (1996) Unruptured tubal pregnancy: local low-dose therapy with methotrexate under trans-vaginal ultrasonographic guidance. *Gynecol Obstet Invest* 41: 76–81

34 Mesogitis SA, Daskalakis GJ, Antsaklis AJ, Papantoniou NE, Papageorgiou JS, Michalas SK (1998) Local application of methotrexate for ectopic pregnancy with a percutaneous puncturing technique. *Gynecol Obstet Invest* 45: 154–158

35 Pisarska MD, Carson SA, Buster JE (1998) Ectopic pregnancy. *Lancet* 351: 1115–1120

36 Yankowitz J, Leake J, Huggins G, Gazaway P, Gates E (1990) Cervical ectopic pregnancy: review of the literature and report of a case treated by single-dose methotrexate therapy. *Obstet Gynecol Surv* 45: 405–414

37 Sonmez AS, Kafkasli A, Balat O, Sarac K, Uryan I, Turhan O, Aydin NE (1994) Cervical pregnancy: can age and parity be predisposing factors? *Acta Obstet Gynecol Scand* 73: 734–736

38 Dall P, Pfisterer J, du Bois A, Wilhelm C, Pfleiderer A (1994) Therapeutic strategies in cervical pregnancy. *Eur J Obstet Gynecol Reprod Biol* 56: 195–200

39 Timor-Tritsch IE, Monteagudo A, Mandeville EO, Peisner DB, Anaya GP, Pirrone EC (1994) Successful management of viable cervical pregnancy by local injection of methotrexate guided by transvaginal ultrasonography. *Am J Obstet Gynecol* 170: 737–739

40 Sherer DM (1990) Treatment of cervical pregnancy with methotrexate. *Am J Obstet Gynecol* 163: 693–694

41 Centini G, Rosignoli L, Severi FM (1994) A case of cervical pregnancy. *Am J Obstet Gynecol* 171: 272–273

42 Ginsburg ES, Frates MC, Rein MS, Fox JH, Hornstein MD, Friedman AJ (1994) Early diagnosis and treatment of cervical pregnancy in an *in vitro* fertilization program. *Fertil Steril* 61: 966–969

43 Monteagudo A, Tarricone NJ, Timor-Tritsch IE, Lerner JP (1996) Successful transvaginal ultrasound-guided puncture and injection of a cervical pregnancy in a patient with simultaneous intrauterine pregnancy and a history of a previous cervical pregnancy. *Ultrasound Obstet Gynecol* 8: 381–386

44 Jurkovic D, Hacket E, Campbell S (1996) Diagnosis and treatment of early cervical pregnancy: a review and a report of two cases treated conservatively. *Ultrasound Obstet Gynecol* 8: 373–380

45 Timor-Tritsch IE, Monteagudo A, Matera C, Veit CR (1992) Sonographic evolution of cornual pregnancies treated without surgery. *Obstet Gynecol* 79: 1044–1049

46 Benifla JL, Fernandez H, Sebban E, Darai E, Frydman R, Madelenat P (1996) Alternative to surgery of treatment of unruptured interstitial pregnancy: 15 cases of medical treatment. *Eur J Obstet Gynecol Reprod Biol* 70: 151–156

47 Baker VL, Givens CR, Cadieux MC (1997) Transvaginal reduction of an interstitial heterotopic pregnancy with preservation of the intrauterine gestation. *Am J Obstet Gynecol* 176: 1384–1385

Index